Guiding Autobiography
Groups for Older Adults

Also of Interest in This Series:

William Halsey Barker, M.D., *Adding Life to Years: Organized Geriatrics Services in Great Britain and Implications for the United States*

Uriel Cohen and Gerald D. Weisman, *Holding On to Home: Designing Environments for People with Dementia*

Dorothy H. Coons, ed., *Specialized Dementia Care Units*

Carl Eisdorfer, Ph.D., M.D., David A. Kessler, M.D., J.D., and Abby N. Spector, M.M.H.S., eds., *Caring for the Elderly: Reshaping Health Policy*

Madelon Lubin Finkel and Hirsch S. Ruchlin, *The Health Care Benefits of Retirees*

Nancy L. Mace, ed., *Dementia Care: Patient, Family, and Community*

William G. Weissert, Jennifer M. Elston, Elise J. Bolda, William N. Zelman, Elizabeth Mutran, and Anne B. Mangum, *Adult Day Care: Findings from a National Survey*

Guiding Autobiography Groups for Older Adults

Exploring the Fabric of Life

James E. Birren and
Donna E. Deutchman

The Johns Hopkins University Press
Baltimore and London

The Johns Hopkins University Press
701 West 40th Street
Baltimore, Maryland 21211
The Johns Hopkins Press Ltd., London

The paper used in this book meets the minimum requirements of
American National Standards for Information Sciences—
Permanence of Paper for Printed Library Materials, ANSI
Z39.48–1984.

Library of Congress Cataloging-in-Publication Data

Birren, James E.
    Guiding autobiography groups for older adults : exploring the
fabric of life / James E. Birren and Donna E. Deutchman.
        p.   cm. — (The Johns Hopkins series in contemporary
medicine and public health)
    Includes bibliographical references.
    Includes index.
    ISBN 0-8018-4161-5 (alk. paper)   ISBN 0-8018-4213 (pbk.)
    1. Autobiography—Therapeutic use.   2. Aged—
Rehabilitation.   3. Self-help groups.   I. Deutchman, Donna E.
II. Title.   III. Series.
    [DNLM: 1. Autobiography.   2. Persuasive Communication—
in old age.   3. Self Concept—in old age.   4. Self-Help
Groups.   5. Writing. BF 697 B619g]
RC953.5.B57   1991
362.1'9897—dc20
DNLM/DLC
for Library of Congress   90-15625

Contents

Foreword, by Robert N. Butler   vii
Preface   ix

1. Strengthening the Fabric of Life   1
   The Therapeutic Role of Guided Autobiography   3
   Contributing to Human Development   4
   Integration and Fulfillment   6
   Contributing to the Family   17
   Contributing to Cognitive Functioning   19
   Releasing Motivation   19
   Adapting to New Roles in the Later Years   20
   Reconciling Life and Accepting Death   22

2. Leading a Guided Autobiography Group   23
   The Guided Autobiography Process   24
   Leadership for a Guided Autobiography Group   25
   Creating the Group   30
   Fostering Group Participation   35
   The Logistics of Meetings   37

3. The Healing Power of the Group   44
   Developmental Exchange   44
   Mutual Acceptance and Support   48
   Interpersonal Relations   49
   Social Gains for Older Adults   54
   So, Why Write?   57

4. The Importance of Guiding Themes   59
    Emotional Saliency and Life Themes   60
    The Use of Sensitizing Questions   63

5. Successful Themes and Sensitizing Questions   67

6. Encouraging Creativity and Divergent Thinking   80
    Creativity and the Older Adult   81
    Conquering the Fear of Writing   82
    The Use of Self-descriptive Words   84
    The Use of Metaphors   86
    The Use of Poetry   88
    Experimenting with Other Senses   90
    The Use of Puppets   92

7. Mastering Potential Obstacles in the Group Process   93
    Overenrollment   93
    Counterproductive Group Members   94
    Signs of Depression and What to Do   98
    Ensuring Institutional Support   100

8. The Next Steps after Guided Autobiography   103
    A Continuous Search for Meaning   104
    Exploring Publishing Interest and Potential   107
    Other Writing Experiences   107
    Creating a Legacy   110
    Guided Autobiography and Medusa's Head   111

9. A Professional's Guide to the Literature, and Implications for
   Future Research   114
    Who Writes Autobiographies?   114
    The Uses of Autobiographical Accounts in Research   120
    The Current Uses and Potential for Future Research   126

References   133
Index   139

Foreword

I BELIEVE that at least four great categories of fitness become more and more essential to maintain as we grow older. The first, and the one we are most familiar with, is physical fitness—the bodily strength, resilience, and agility that are stimulated by appropriate exercise. Intellectual fitness, the second category, comes from keeping the mind engaged and active. The third, social fitness, requires forming and maintaining significant personal relationships that may be called upon in good times and in bad. No less important is the fourth category, purpose fitness. Purpose fitness means having feelings of self-esteem and control over one's own life. There are many ways to cultivate these feelings, but writing an autobiography may be the best of all.

Through the process of shaping our life story, we learn about ourselves—where we have been, where we are now, and, it is to be hoped, where we are going. Although writing one's autobiography may not be considered a form of therapy per se, there is no question that it can help us discover our strengths and weaknesses and come to terms with the lives we have led.

Reviewing their past helps individuals feel that their lives have had meaning and purpose. Furthermore, it helps them resolve continuing or resurgent conflicts, reconcile internal contradictions, overcome problems, and master complicated feelings or relationships with loved ones. Last, but not least, autobiography becomes a cherished legacy to younger generations.

But faced with a blank sheet of paper and an assignment to write about their lives, many people feel overwhelmed by the enormity of the task: Where should they begin? What should they include or leave out? How deeply should the various life experiences be examined? A strong argument can be made for enlisting the assistance of a knowledgeable guide to lead the process. *Guiding Autobiography Groups for Older Adults: Exploring the Fabric of Life* shows the reader how to become such a leader. Drawing on Dr. Birren's many years of experience with guided autobiographies, the authors have written a definitive manual for people who plan to conduct autobiography groups in a variety of settings: nursing homes, senior centers, and community centers, to name just a few.

That the authors' prescription for effective autobiography writing includes group interaction is significant, particularly for older people, who often become isolated as a result of changing life circumstances. Writing groups provide participants with opportunities to develop new relationships and combat loneliness. In addition, the group's support, acceptance, and insights can help solidify the therapeutic value of autobiography writing. This book thoroughly covers the intricacies of running a group, underscoring its benefits and troubleshooting its possible pitfalls.

An important function of the group leader is to facilitate autobiography writing. To help, the authors suggest and discuss the use of themes in guiding the writing process. Writing in response to themes presented by the group leader gives participants a shared basis and language for their work and helps them focus on the most significant crossroads in their lives.

Guiding Autobiography Groups for Older Adults: Exploring the Fabric of Life is a most welcome addition to the growing body of literature on the relevance of autobiography or life review in the later years. It will no doubt stimulate readers to establish autobiography groups of their own in whatever setting they find themselves. And because of the good advice the book offers, they will become effective group leaders, much to the benefit of the older participants, who will discover the many rewards of recapturing the past.

Robert N. Butler, m.d.
Brookdale Professor and Chairman
Department of Geriatrics and Adult Development
Mount Sinai School of Medicine

Preface

WRITING about one's life and sharing it with others is a high point of human experience that should be encouraged by those who can take the initiative and provide the time and energy to guide the process.

As a guided autobiography group leader, you can create an environment that provides social support and mental stimulation for older adults to review their life stories and share them with others. Using strategies that ensure a positive group experience and sensitize group members to the critical themes around which our lives are patterned, you can help older adults develop a heightened sense of self-awareness, social acceptance, and self-esteem. For many older adults, life changes such as widowhood and retirement can damage feelings of identity and self-worth. Guided autobiography is ideally suited to foster in the older adult a belief that his or her life is meaningful and something of which to be proud.

We have written this book in response to the many telephone calls and letters we have received requesting information on how to create and conduct guided autobiography groups. Requests have come from people who provide assistance to older adults through organizations such as senior centers, mental health care facilities, and community centers; from counselors, social workers, and activities directors in nursing homes and other long-term care facilities; from people seeking meaningful ways to assist inmates in women's prisons and other persons who might benefit from reviewing the life events and choices that have led them to their current circumstances; and from older adults who would like to engage in the process along with friends and family. We designed this book to help you conduct guided autobiography groups that can promote well-being, develop friendships, and create increased feelings of self-efficacy in older adults.

After helping hundreds of people write their autobiographies, the most important thing that we have learned confirms Hemingway's observation that "the world breaks everyone and afterward, many are stronger at the broken places." Each group realizes that people are all survivors. In reviewing the details of their lives and experiencing the support of the group, people become impressed with how much they, themselves, have survived, and the many ways they have been tested by events and by people.

Since the first course, more than fourteen years ago, the guided autobiography process has been presented with a variety of perspectives and goals, from academic, to social, to personal. It has been presented as a course, as a workshop, as a group process, and as an informal support group. It has been presented over the course of eleven weeks (meeting once a week), as a three-day-long workshop, and in as many ways as about twenty hours can be combined. It has been offered in the United States, Canada, Germany, Korea, the Netherlands, and Japan. It has always been met with the enthusiasm of participants and resulted in positive outcomes for both the group members and group leaders.

This book has been written to extend guided autobiography to an audience beyond the scope of the current authors. This process can be adapted in a number of ways to help the many different individuals who can benefit from a guided review of their lives and group interactions.

To provide the opportunity for older adults to strengthen their identities through recording and sharing their life stories is in itself a gratifying experience. For some, the experience will lead to a written legacy for their families and others. To observe the coming alive of old memories and emotions, and the revitalization of power and meaning in life, can be extremely satisfying for all participants in the guided autobiography group process. It is our belief that through this process you can help older adults come to terms with their lives as they have been led and meet new demands and life changes with increased confidence and competence.

We wish to express our appreciation to those colleagues who reviewed early drafts of our manuscript and provided helpful comments: Benjamin Gottlieb from the University of Guelph, Barbara Haight from the College of Nursing of the University of South Carolina, James Magee of the College of New Rochelle, Erdman Palmore from Duke University, Edmund Sherman from the Ringel Institute of Gerontology, and V. Quinton Wacks, Jr., from Lincoln Memorial University. Special thanks to Jean Lesher, whose early input helped focus our efforts.

Guiding Autobiography Groups for Older Adults

Chapter 1

Strengthening the Fabric of Life

YOU CAN HELP older adults build greater understanding and self-worth by leading guided autobiography groups. From the viewpoint of human development, there is little of greater importance to each of us than gaining a perspective on our own life story, to find, clarify, and deepen meaning in the accumulated experience of a lifetime (Butler, 1963; Hall, 1922; Myerhoff and Tufte, 1975; Sarbin, 1986). Particularly in the later years, a person needs to believe that his or her life has mattered, that it has had a purpose or an impact on the world. Guided autobiography enhances these feelings, promotes successful adaptation to old age, and assists positive choices by persons at a crossroad in life. A grasp of the fabric of one's life can make a significant contribution to well-being in later life. When it results in a written form, it can also create an important legacy for families.

Guided autobiography is designed to combine individual and group experiences with autobiography, incorporating (1) group interaction and leadership to sensitize people to the overlooked and unappreciated past and to generate new perspectives on the issues of their lives; (2) private reflection and the writing of two-page life stories on selected life themes; and (3) reading these life stories and sharing thoughts in a mutually encouraging group, moderated by a group leader.

Guided autobiography is based on a number of concepts about how people develop understanding of themselves and their lives and how memory, personal reflection, and present perceptions interact. It evokes and guides reminiscence, that is, the recall of events from the past, and directs the individuals to examine their memories from the perspective of the present. It is a form of semistructured life review, bringing review of events and emotions over the life course one step further—into a group context wherein different members' perceptions and histories can evoke further reflection and challenge earlier views of the self.

Other reminiscence and life-review techniques have evolved around different principles. Life review, as initiated by Butler (1963) and Lewis (1973), emphasizes the evocative aspects of the end of life. Butler viewed proximity to death as a stimulus to the resurgence of old memories and conflicts that need resolution. In its original form, it did not involve the group process or the suggestion of themes by a group leader or therapist. Similarly, reminiscence techniques (e.g., Ingersoll and Silverman, 1978; Kaminsky, 1978) utilize spontaneous and free-flowing memories and may or may not be used in a group context.

Guided autobiography is an efficient way for older adults to review their lives by following a proven series of evocative themes and responding to questions designed to promote reflection. The group leader uses the themes and sensitizing questions to guide persons interested in developing greater awareness of themselves through an organized recall of memories and emotions. The themes are presented and discussed sequentially so that the recollections and their interpretation can be woven into a picture of the individual life course and an integrated understanding of the fabric of a life. The sensitizing questions elaborate on potential contents of or approaches to the themes.

Sharing life stories with other group members also refreshes one's memories of the neglected past. It (1) reinforces and sustains the motivation to review life, (2) allows individuals to reexperience parts of themselves in the stories of others, and (3) provides a context for the development of new friendships.

In guided autobiography, participants are asked to write and share with the group a series of brief autobiographical life stories based on assigned themes. The guided autobiography group meets a minimum of ten times for at least two hours each time. Sessions consist of a discussion of the next meeting's theme, to be written in advance of that meeting, and members' reading and discussing the life stories written at home on the theme assigned for the current day.

Members write and share with the group nine brief, two-page, autobiographical life accounts. A typical sequence of assignments might include writing one's life histories on the following themes:

1. The major branching points in my life
2. My family
3. My career or major life work
4. The role of money in my life

5. My health and body image
6. The loves and hates over my lifetime
7. My sexual identity, sex roles, and sexual experiences
8. My experiences with death and ideas about dying
9. The history of my aspirations and life goals and the meaning of my life

The Therapeutic Role of Guided Autobiography

Guided autobiography is not designed to be used as formal therapy since it is not actively directed toward the cure or amelioration of a disease or a social or emotional problem. It does, however, have therapeutic value as a by-product that occurs naturally.

The term *therapeutic* is defined as "having healing powers" (Webster's Third New International Dictionary, 1981). Many things are therapeutic without being therapy per se. They are distinguished from therapy in that they do not directly or actively pursue change in behavior or emotions, although positive changes may result. For example, the following can be described as therapeutic but would not be viewed as forms of therapy:

- Exercise that is not prescribed by a health care professional
- Friendships
- Relaxation time
- Confidant relationships
- Gardening
- Playing a musical instrument

Not unlike these other activities that have therapeutic qualities, guided autobiography has "healing powers" resulting from the reconciliation of longstanding issues. Reviewing the history of a life in the context of the present self and in a supportive group affords insight. As such, guided autobiography can be employed by nontherapeutically oriented professionals and nonprofessionals.

Guided autobiography represents an important service to:

1. Older adults, offering an opportunity to develop greater meaning in life and increased feelings of competency and worth.

2. Those confronted by difficult transitions in life, such as,

   - widowhood
   - career change or entrance into the work force

- retirement
- divorce
- transition to a childless household
- moving to a nursing home or hospice

It places these transitions into the broader context of the entire life span, helping the individual to gain confidence and put current concerns into the perspective of challenges already met.

3. Those adapting to recent disability, who are often in need of emotional support, pragmatic advice, and reassurance that they are competent to meet new demands.

4. Those who must change their life-styles to maintain health and increase productivity, for example,

- recovering heart attack victims
- substance abusers

5. All persons seeking greater understanding and acceptance of themselves.

Contributing to Human Development

In the remainder of this chapter, we will explore the human developmental advantages of conducting guided autobiography groups for older adults and the related emotional and pragmatic gains. Our conclusions grow out of research to assess the consequences of life review and the autobiographical process, a form of which is guided autobiography. Research has helped to clarify important outcomes and to highlight benefits for mature adults. Table 1-1 summarizes some of this research.

The findings summarized in Table 1-1 have been supported by follow-up comments and letters of older adults who have joined in guided autobiography since its inception. These people have reported the following positive outcomes:

- Sense of increased personal power and importance
- Recognition of past adaptive strategies and application to current needs and problems
- Reconciliation with the past and resolution of past resentments and negative feelings
- Resurgence of interest in past activities or hobbies
- Development of friendships with other group members

Table 1-1. Benefits of Life Review/Autobiography: An Overview of the Research

Area of Benefit	Focus of Study/Article	Author(s)
Acceptance of death	Dying persons	Georgemiller and Maloney, 1984
Cognitive functioning	Older adults	Hughston and Merriam, 1982
Coping/adaptation	Sheltered housing residents	Coleman, 1974
Depression (relief from)	Demented older adults	Goldwasser, Auerbach, and Harkins, 1987
	Older adults	Magee, 1988
Ego integrity	Older adult males	Boylin, Gordon, and Nehrke, 1976 Havighurst and Glaser, 1972
Fulfillment	Older adults	Buhler and Massarik, 1968
Future orientation	Older adults	Costa and Kastenbaum, 1967
Increased sense of continuity	Older adults	Myerhoff and Tufte, 1975
Integration	Older adults	Butler, 1963
Intergenerational connectedness	Older adults	Greene, 1982 Myerhoff and Tufte, 1975
Meaning in life	All ages	Birren and Hedlund, 1987
	Older adults	Lewis and Butler, 1974
Memory capacity	Older adults	Ebersole, 1978
Mental adaptability	Nursing home residents	Berghorn and Schafer, 1987
Reconciliation or resolution of past	Older adults	Birren and Hedlund, 1987
Role clarity/transition	Older adults	Greene, 1982
Self-disclosure	All ages	Birren and Hedlund, 1987
Self-esteem	All ages Older adults	Allport, 1942 Butler, 1967 Ebersole, 1978
Self-understanding	All ages Adults	Annis, 1967 Hately, 1985
Social integration	Older adults	Ebersole, 1978
Spiritual well-being	Adults	Hately, 1985

- Greater sense of meaning in life
- Ability to face the nearing end of life with a feeling that one has contributed to the world

Such outcomes are the goals of professionals and others who seek to increase competence and confidence in older adults. The method of guided autobiography is a valuable tool for professionals in the areas of counseling, nursing, psychiatry, psychology, adult education, rehabilitation, senior center administration, and social work, among others.

Integration and Fulfillment

The opportunity to integrate or make sense of one's life as it has been lived in relation to how it might have been lived is important for most older adults. Most older adults need to reconcile past values and goals with present realities. Elements of the task of reconciliation are also seen at other periods of transition, such as upon leaving school, making a job change, entering into retirement, or when the last child leaves home. These issues, however, are most meaningful in the second half of life or near the end of life, when the future, and therefore opportunities for altering the life course, are perceived as limited. Then, guided autobiography offers a chance for the older adult to:

- Reconcile the way a life has been lived
- Clarify and supply details of the legacy and image he or she wishes to leave behind
- Modify plans and choose new activities
- Reaffirm the value of the past and derive a feeling of fulfillment in life

Older adults are ripe for guided autobiography, and it is especially beneficial for them since contemporary society in general does not provide the opportunity for the old to review and tell their life stories. Situations must be created so that such opportunities can be provided.

In guided autobiography, older adults recall and relive a wide range of personal experiences and become aware of the various aspects of their lives. Often, feelings of significance are derived not from rediscovery or reappraisal of a single major experience but rather from reviewing the life course as a whole—discovering the cumulative experiences and what they add up to. In summing up the experiences of a lifetime, people are frequently surprised by their ability to have survived and transcended many difficult times. Reactions of the group often support a person's perception of transitions as arduous and provide a sense that he or she showed the ability to overcome formidable hardships of life.

This brings to mind a scene from Ron Howard's contemporary film *Parenthood,* which focuses on a four-generation family. The matriarch of the family spends much of the film silently observing the struggles of her grandchildren. Her sole advice is given in the form of a metaphor based on a review of her own life. She likens some lives to a roller coaster and others to a merry-go-round. She notes that the latter may be safer but that she finds greater satisfaction in the former. The roller coaster not only is more interesting but also provides a greater sense of self-worth as the ups and downs of life are reviewed and the ability to transcend is revealed.

You'll Know Better Where You're Going Because You'll Know Where You've Been

Renewed confidence in one's capacity to adapt, along with increased understanding of one's personal agenda, can form the basis for successful future choices. The insight of the group leader and other group members can facilitate the process of expanding appreciation and understanding of the self. Through the use of themes and sensitizing questions, the group leader can guide older adults in reviewing the past, to achieve better understanding of what has worked for them. This is seen in the following example:

Mary entered a guided autobiography group partly in the hope that the group leader would help with a decision about a new home. Mary currently lived with her husband in the same house in which they had raised their three children. They had lived there for more than thirty years; and although it was too large for two people, they remained there so that they had ample room for grandchildren to visit.

Now, Mary was confronted with the need to adjust to her new role as primary caregiver to a husband with Alzheimer's disease. It was increasingly difficult for her to keep up with her housework, and the two-floor layout caused problems due to her husband's night wandering. She now questioned whether she should attempt to sell the house and enter a life care community that would provide assistance for her husband if she, herself, should become ill. She was burdened by uncertainty regarding the financial commitment and the feeling that this would represent failure in providing care to her family.

In completing the theme assignment on the history of her life's work, Mary recounted many instances in which she had helped her husband in his business. A number of group members pointed out that she demonstrated keen decision making, which resulted in financial successes. This gave Mary greater confidence in her ability to take on new financial responsibilities.

In addition, a life-story essay of another group member brought Mary a new awareness of the importance of seeking assistance rather than attempting to do everything herself. The group leader's comment about similarities in the two life stories led Mary to begin to recognize in her own history a desire to control all aspects of her family's health and safety. She recognized the importance of allowing herself to depend on others in the care of her husband.

The admiration expressed by the group about the way she had lived her life, coupled with reawakened memories of ways in which she had supported her husband throughout their lives together, gave Mary greater appreciation of her contribution to her husband's life.

Mary decided to enlist the assistance of her children in making the final decision about her next step, but she completed guided autobiography with an increased view of her self-worth.

As this example illustrates, the autobiographical process can be viewed as a method of taking inventory of the events that shaped one's life and recounting the decision strategies, skills, and strengths shown during a long life. This personal inventory can be tested against the views expressed by others in the group and used to develop a map for future action.

Just as an inventory of successful strategies can provide increased confidence in meeting new demands, an understanding of how chance events have helped to shape the life course can have a freeing quality. Particularly for those who experience a sense of failure and regret, insight into the influencing factors that are out of their control can help focus attention on adaptive capacities and strength in the face of hardship. The guided autobiography group and its leader can help members identify aspects of their lives about which they should not be experiencing a sense of blame or failure.

Strengthening Concepts of the Self

The writing and sharing of your life story leads to a stronger identity, a grasp of who you are. To describe your identity, it is necessary to specify the elements of the self and how, as an individual, you differ from others. Participating in guided autobiography can strengthen identity, afford a better grasp of the details of identity, and lead to a new evaluation of the enduring self.

Identity involves an evaluation not only of *who* you are but also of *what* you are, an assessment of your personal attributes, such as good-bad, desirable-undesirable, and kind-cruel. Choices of these attributes and their criteria are highly personal and based on your expectations of who and what a person should be. For example, one person's identity might be as a man, leading to an elaboration of what kind of man: strong-weak, reliable-irresponsible, ambitious-lazy. Another man might evaluate himself on different attributes, such as wealthy-poor, successful-unsuccessful, powerful-powerless.

The self-descriptive words we use tell much about our sense of identity. Research on self-descriptive words reveals that, although highly personal, there are common characteristics in the ways in which persons identify themselves. For example, a study by Birren, Hoppe, and Birren (unpublished) of 363 participants in guided autobiography revealed 17 words most frequently used by persons in describing themselves. In this study, subjects were asked to write a list of words that best described themselves. They were then asked to number these words, with the first being most descriptive of their identity. Table 1-2 provides a list of the 17 most frequently used self-descriptive words and specifies the number of persons who chose each word as the first, second, or third most relevant.

The five most commonly used descriptive words were *friendly, intelligent, loving, sensitive,* and *caring.* The diversity in words is impressive. The most common first word was *friendly,* although only 18 of 363 people chose it. We may conclude that identity is a very individualistic matter. It should also be noted that the commonly chosen descriptive words are largely behavioral characteristics, not physical attributes.

Further insight into an individual's self-evaluation might be inferred from the types of self-descriptive words used, that is, nouns, verbs, adjectives, and adverbs, as well as the relationships they imply and the positive or negative connotations. It is both interesting and enlightening for guided autobiography group members to do this exercise before and after the entire series of meetings and the writing and sharing of their life stories. The

Table 1-2. High Frequency Self-descriptive Words
(in alphabetical order)

Words	First Choice	Second Choice	Third Choice
Active	6	7	0
Caring	13	0	0
Concerned	8	0	0
Creative	7	0	0
Curious	8	8	0
Energetic	6	0	0
Friendly	18	12	0
Happy	8	0	0
Inquisitive	6	0	0
Intelligent	7	13	13
Loving	11	7	10
Male	1	0	0
Optimistic	6	0	0
Responsible	6	0	6
Sensitive	12	9	7
Woman	7	0	0

changes in how members choose to describe and thereby evaluate themselves give a sense of closure to the experience. (For more on this topic, see "Use of Self-descriptive Words," Chapter 6.)

The Construction of Identity

Each person constructs an identity based on analyses of the differences in three versions of the self: (1) the *real* self as defined by personal interpretation of the actual self, (2) the *ideal* self, a model of the "perfect" self, the person he or she would like to be, and (3) the *social-image* self, a person's perception of how other people view him or her. It could be argued that self-esteem arises from an evaluation of the difference between the real and ideal selves; while self-efficacy, the feeling that you are competent and can have the impact you seek, is measured by the congruency between the ideal self and the social-image self. Self-actualization, satisfaction with who you are and a feeling of fulfillment from what you have accomplished, might then be viewed as determined by the distance between these three selves, with the greatest degree of self-actualization obtained by those whose ideal, real, and social-image selves converge (see Fig. 1-1).

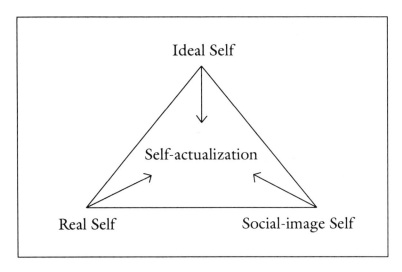

Figure 1-1. Emergence of self-actualization

A large difference among the three images of the self creates tension and discomfort. Alternatively, a high level of similarity of the images is accompanied by contentment and security in relation to others. Guided autobiography helps to clarify and reduce the difference between the ideal and actual selves and exposes the social image to scrutiny and review. The guided autobiography group acts as a mirror of the social self, while at the same time presenting an opportunity to compare openly and to contrast a person's perception of the real and ideal selves with how others see him or her. It provides unique insight into how different each person's ideal self is, putting the goals we set for ourselves into a new perspective. The group leader can promote the development of such insight by asking group members to provide feedback on statements that reflect a given member's self-view. The result is greater understanding, an increased sense of importance, and feelings of support and mastery. The following is an example of how this came about for one group member:

> When the group leader began a discussion on the development of self-concept (derived from the discussion above), Penny began to see that her own self-esteem was greatly diminished by constant assessment of the large difference between her real and ideal selves. Penny explained to the group that she had constructed an ideal self based on a "heroine" from her early youth,

a friend of the family who had served as a role model throughout Penny's life. Penny characterized this woman as intelligent, competent in all circumstances, popular and attractive, and she strove to emulate her. Penny's poor self-view was based on her opinion that she always fell short of this ideal model.

The group leader encouraged Penny to reconstruct her memory of this woman from the perspective of an adult. Penny recalled life circumstances that had placed the woman in a unique leadership role for her time, and she realized that the woman had met many challenges but had also been defeated by some. In reviewing these circumstances with the group and now as an adult, Penny recognized that the real woman actually fell short of Penny's ideal. Penny began to realize that much of her ideal was based on a childlike, and indeed childhood, interpretation of events. She began to develop a more realistic version of her ideal self and, in turn, achieved a greater sense of her own worth and power.

As demonstrated in Penny's experience, by reviewing her self-evaluative concepts with the group, the guided autobiography group leader can bring to awareness factors that influence definitions of the real, ideal, and social-image selves. This opens the door for further contemplation of these ideas and, potentially, resolution or reduction of the distance between them.

Resolution of differences among the three selves is important for all mature adults. These aspects of the self are developed during childhood, with greatest influence by the outer world and how others, particularly parents, view who and how the child should be. Adolescence is generally the period during which the person perceives the greatest degree of distance between who they are, who they would like to be, and how they are viewed by others. It is marked by a dual focus on developing a sense of individuality while at the same time seeking social acceptance. During this period, peers are paramount in determining the social-image and ideal selves and their differences.

In keeping with the developmental theories of such renowned scholars as Charlotte Buhler, Erik Erikson, Daniel Levinson, and Roger Gould, later adulthood, beginning around age 50, is a time for integration—resolution and acceptance of one's identity being key to mental and emotional well-being. Some middle-aged and older adults continue to experience insecurities characteristic of earlier stages of human development, that is, past tensions and discomforts about how they fit into the world. This means that the distances among the three selves are overblown by the individual, resulting in a feeling that one has failed. Guided autobiography can play a vital role in freeing these feelings, leading to resolution.

Reedy and Birren (1980) studied forty-five members in guided autobiography before and after participating in the process. These group members completed a battery of four psychological tests designed to measure the effects of guided autobiography on self-concept, ideal self, social-image self, self-acceptance, social acceptance, mood, and anxiety. Sixty percent of those studied showed greater self-acceptance or personal integration as measured by the Leary Interpersonal Checklist (see Fig. 1-2). Older adults showed more change toward self-acceptance as compared to

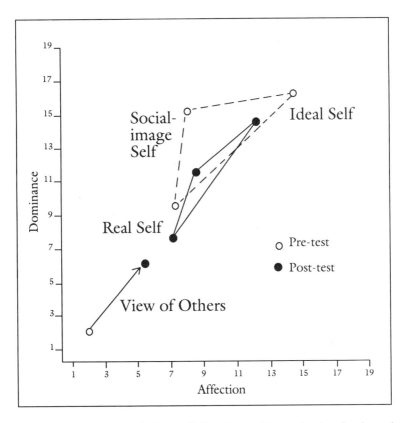

Figure 1-2. Mean scores before and after the autobiography class for the real, ideal, and social-image selves and for the view of others, as measured by the Leary Interpersonal Checklist (adapted from Reedy and Birren, 1980)

other guided autobiography participants, "suggesting that Guided Autobiography, while helpful at any age, may be most beneficial for older adults." In short, the data suggested that guided autobiography has "an anti-depressant effect by (1) increasing self-acceptance and personal integration; (2) reducing anxiety and tension; (3) increasing feelings of energy and vigor; and (4) increasing social connectedness and the capacity for rewarding interpersonal relationships" (Reedy and Birren, 1980, poster session).

Related research by distinguished psychologists such as Boylin, Gordon, and Nehrke (1976); Costa and Kastenbaum (1967); and Elbaz (1988) also supports this view. A positive relationship has been found between the amount of reminiscence and the degree of ego-integrity (or self-integration) achieved. Here, reminiscence is defined as the process of recalling the events of one's past, a process upon which the more structured guided autobiography is built. It is important to note that the relationship between reminiscence and ego-integrity, and the positive outcome it implies for self-acceptance, is found even when the memories of past experiences are painful or negative.

Maintaining a Sense of Continuity

Guided autobiography reveals ways in which a person has maintained continuity throughout life. Continuity, particularly as it concerns a person's belief system and related patterns of behavior, reaffirms and supports a coherent sense of self. If a person is able to affirm and accept the contents of life and the continuity of identity, the late-life task of integration is advanced. This requires that one take responsibility for one's life, while at the same time locating it within the cultural and social climate that helped to determine its progression. The members' life stories that are similar because of shared social history and events can provide insight in this area. The group leader can promote integration by applying the strategies discussed in Chapter 3.

Awareness of self-continuity provides a feeling of security and inner strength that can greatly enhance one's sense of meaning in life. Awareness of continuity also supports self-esteem in times of stress.

Mark participated in an evening guided autobiography group at his local church. He was referred to this group when he was confronted at age 64 with the need to adjust to a new life as a divorced grandfather. Mark reported to the group that his greatest anxiety about his impending divorce concerned his relationship with his adult son (a widower) and his grandchildren.

In his autobiography, Mark wrote that after the death of his daughter-in-law, his wife began to babysit the grandchildren each day after school. Since his own retirement a year ago, Mark also had become involved in raising these two young girls. Despite his daily participation in their upbringing, Mark held the view that the primary care was provided by his soon-to-be ex-wife. He told the group that he was worried that his connection to the girls would weaken as a result of his divorce, but he was anxious about caring for them on his own.

In discussing his life story, the group leader pointed out that Mark had relayed a history of relationships in which he served as mentor, both in his career as a teacher and in his private life. Through the group process, Mark began to see his role as mentor as connected to an ability to nurture others, a personality trait he had not clearly identified up until that time. He traced this as far back as he could remember and recalled how he had a love for animals as a boy.

With the group leader's assistance in tracing this ability and desire to care for others beyond the scope of his marriage, Mark began to develop a sense of continuity of this facet of his personality. This, and his growing relationships with others in the group, helped Mark build confidence in his ability to demonstrate this behavior without the support of his wife.

After a loss, an essential part of the healing process is the discovery that despite new circumstances, you are still yourself. Guided autobiography assists this process by focusing attention on the entire life span, helping the group member recall who and how he was prior to the attachment that had recently been severed, in this case, the marriage. Table 1-3 provides examples of such losses and how a focus on continuity can aid in the process of adaptation.

Cultural and Ethnic Identity in a Changing Society

As our society becomes increasingly diverse ethnically, issues of cultural and ethnic identity and their role in mental health become more and more important. Acceptance of one's heritage and the need to "connect" with ancestors and especially with parents and grandparents can represent

Table 1-3. Continuity and Adaptation to Loss

Loss	Continuity	Adaptive Potential	Impact on Adjustment
Divorce	Behavior/ personality	Nurturant behavior	New investment in relationships beyond the marriage
Widowhood	Behavior	Ability to manage a household and hold leadership roles in the community	Confidence to enter the work force
	Belief system	Reliance on religion/ spirituality	Ability to cope with loss and to focus on devoting self to God's will
Retirement	Behavior/ personality	Ability to adjust to shifting roles and to engage in entrepreneurial endeavors	Shift to productive role in a volunteer capacity
Disability	Belief system	Focus on charity and spiritual well-being of others	Ability to cope with loss through revision of the self-view to emphasize inner strength
	Behavior	Innovative strategies employed throughout life	Confidence in the ability to compensate for loss
Change of residence	Behavior	Community involvement	Joining residents' council and making new friendships

major influences in the development of self-esteem. Guided autobiography can engender a greater understanding of the role ethnicity has played in development. It is a fertile ground for exploring the development of values and meaning in life.

The use of guided autobiography among older adults with similar ethnic and cultural backgrounds provides a rich environment for reliving and translating into the current context aspects of ethnicity that were and are particularly enjoyable. For example, "heritage groups" have been formed in long-term care settings, promoting examination of personal history in the context of recalling a shared cultural history and ancestry (Price, 1983). Such groups provide an opportunity not only to reminisce but also to share the past through the use of old photographs, music, and memorabilia. Such tangible reminders serve to stimulate the memory, leading participants to recall aspects of their personal histories that might otherwise remain buried.

The group leader can facilitate this aspect of guided autobiography by providing an environment in which ethnic differences are openly discussed and greeted with acceptance and support (see section on group rules in Chapter 2). This can be a unifying experience to celebrate ethnic differences together. This might be done in the form of a potluck lunch, in which each person brings a food typical of his or her cultural heritage. Or, pictures might be brought and shared with the group that depict family or ancestors in regional dress.

Contributing to the Family

Guided autobiography invariably evokes memories of family episodes and can assist people in seeing "themselves and kin with greater empathy, and using their insight for the benefit of younger generations" (Magee, 1988, p. 17).

In reviewing life, role changes and exchanges with children, parents, and grandparents are revealed. One example of how this can be of benefit is the situation of a midlife husband and wife newly faced with the transition to a childless household. Guided autobiography can bring to mind how the couple interacted early in their marriage, prior to the birth of their first child. They can review the past and recall the shared experiences that helped form the marriage before parenthood. Such memories can assist the couple in redefining their changing partnership.

Explorations of past transitions are relevant not only to the older adult but also to other family members. For example, adult children, faced with an increasingly dependent, older-adult parent, are able to draw on earlier adaptive family experiences related to the transfer of responsibilities and reliance. Not all life changes are easy, with good outcomes. Negative examples can also be used to advantage to portray ways to avoid poor handling of crises and events. Some of our ancestors may have handled situations in particularly poor ways that can lead the current generations to laugh as well as to learn.

Sharing autobiographical writings can provide family members with bridges to historical times they may not have known or understood and assist younger generations in synthesizing their own identities. In this process, older persons represent "living stories" of tradition and transcendence. Sharing of the family history provides a common ground, instilling a sense of belonging and continuity.

Understanding the continuity of a family can free the person of guilt and anger by (1) exposing the roots of family successes, failures, conflicts, and hardships; (2) identifying similarities among family members; and (3) helping a person come to terms with family issues that, in the past, might have been viewed as a fault of another person or oneself. This is seen in the following example:

> Brian wrote, "My great-grandfather was killed by a beer keg dropped from the fourth story window of a corner bar. He was not the only one in my family who died of alcohol, although he was certainly unique in that it killed him from the outside. . . . His greatest contribution was a family metaphor that has lasted for generations."
>
> Brian had always blamed his alcoholic father for dying when he was only four years old. This anger had pervaded many of his relationships over the course of his life and had produced a great deal of anxiety about his own relationship with his son. Through reviewing his family history in the guided autobiography group, Brian was able to come to terms with the enormous role that alcoholism, the disease his father died from, had played throughout his family history.

The group leader's help was in expressing empathy toward Brian's father, enabling Brian to begin to see his father more as victim than as abandoner. The support of the group also helped Brian face the future with renewed confidence in his own capacity to avoid this particular family tradition. This kind of transcendence is often observed in adults who obtain a feeling of greater empowerment once they are able to view their parents as people rather than as censors or omniscient beings, as is seen in the following group members' experiences:

> Marcus achieved a sense of freedom when he wrote and later told the guided autobiography group, "I come from a family of slobs. Even my father's brother cheated him." In such comments the listener and the storyteller grasp the meaning of being a part of such a background, as well as what it means to rise above it.
>
> In another instance, Carol wrote that when she was in high

school her father told her that she was so smart that if she had been a boy he would have sent her to medical school. Now, in retirement, she has reconciled her earlier views with the reality that women can be both feminine and smart—a reality that, in her earlier life, had made her uncertain and ambivalent.

Contributing to Cognitive Functioning

In the past decade, exercise has become a major focus in our society. The public has come to understand that for the body to function at its optimal level, it must be challenged and used regularly. This view is best summarized in the adage, "use it or lose it." The same statement should also be applied to the brain, the most vital organ of the body. Research supports the view that the proper functioning of mental capacity in healthy persons relies on adequate and frequent exercise of cognitive capacity (Willis and Schaie, 1985).

The loss of memory and cognitive capacity is a major concern in the later years of life. Prevention of anxiety about memory loss and amelioration of some memory impairments is a focus in long-term care facilities that seek to maximize residents' potentials and quality of life. Memories provide material that can be used in structuring cognitive activities and stimulating mental ability.

In guided autobiography, a person does not simply remember the facts of his or her past. Memories of prior experiences enter consciousness together with their past and present emotions. These provide material for synthesis and integration of the past with the present, which in turn lead to *planfulness*. Persons with a planning outlook seem to have a more optimistic view of life with less depression (Thomae, 1970). Thus, guided autobiography is useful as an intervention with older adults suffering from cognitive impairment as secondary to, or the result of, depression (Hughston and Merriam, 1982). It is also useful to those suffering from mild dementia, helping to reorient participants to time and place through identifying the past as such. Since some degree of verbal fluency is required to participate in this process, the process is not expected to benefit those suffering from severe dementia.

Releasing Motivation

With increased confidence and morale comes motivation. Group leaders and older adults comment that after participating in the guided autobiography, they become energized. They meet new challenges with a better sense of their own capacities and experience and with greater optimism and vitality. Some of this released motivation is directed at further integrating life experiences, expanding the autobiography to create a family legacy, and planning for the future.

Adapting to New Roles in the Later Years

Taking inventory of the strategies used to successfully navigate changes over the life course is an important resource in the later years, as people are faced with the need to shift roles, often from a productive family provider and leader to a dependent, frail older person. Some of the changes that may be required by later life are the following:

From	*To*
Work force	Retirement
Family provider/income generator	Fixed income and/or financial dependency
Member of couple	Widow(er)
Caregiver	Dependent family member
Health	Frailty
Own home	Institutional care
Producer	Mentor

If past strengths are appreciated, such changes can motivate the older person to develop new, satisfying, and productive roles that fit with current demands and disabilities. New roles for older adults are crucial to our society. These are particularly appropriate for older adults, who have often achieved a greater degree of wisdom. Just a few of these roles include:

Mentor
Consultant
Confidant
Volunteer
Historian
Disseminator of the family legacy
Grandparent or great-grandparent
Second- or third-career member in the work force

Interaction with others in the guided autobiography group can help an older adult explore the potential for new roles. The group leader can stimulate this process by raising the topic of potential roles for discussion and noting trends in research, scholarship, and advocacy which promote such roles as vital contributions by older adults.

Guided autobiography helps in coping with problems of old age in other ways as well. As Kaminsky (1978, p. 30) points out, among other things, it may provide material that leads to a reorganization of personality and a fuller acceptance of one's life cycle; it furthers interpersonal relationships; and it helps older adults cope with grief and depression resulting from personal losses.

New Skills for New Demands

By helping the older adult build confidence in the ability to learn new skills, change can be encouraged through guided autobiography. Physical disability and other age-related concerns can be approached positively, as something to be managed. This perspective is supported by research findings (see Table 1-1): Older persons who engage in guided autobiography are more likely to maintain an orientation toward the future, continuing to plan for future needs and to approach future challenges with mental vitality, as is seen in the following example.

Mike entered a guided autobiography group as part of a company program for pre-retirement planning. Like many of the employees, Mike had derived a large portion of his self-concept from his role as "worker." As a construction worker, he took great pride in his abilities, many of which relied on physical strength and endurance. In recent years, advancing age had limited his role, and eventually resulted in earlier-than-planned retirement. It was now necessary for Mike to redefine his role.

As might be expected, much of Mike's autobiographical writing was approached from his dominating career perspective. But the group leader noted that he was beginning to identify roles outside the scope of physical labor as he recalled the many times he had assisted the "bosses" in strategizing. Other group members also began to identify the more cognitive aspects of his work, for example, solving communication problems between architects and laborers, and to discuss with Mike how they might translate to meaningful future roles.

Adaptation to a Retirement or Nursing Home

In addition to helping adaptation to disability or retirement, the guided autobiography can assist the adjustment in moving to new living environments. It fosters new friendships within the facility, rather than a preoccupation with a sense of loss. Also, constructive reminiscing in a new setting, encouraged by guided autobiography, can decrease feelings of loss, depression, and isolation by focusing attention on positive experiences of the past. Even painful memories can help to decrease depression when we realize that we went on in life and transcended the hardships.

Reconciling Life and Accepting Death

Guided autobiography can be of major benefit to those faced with impending death. It assists older adults and others in developing greater acceptance of death by promoting reconciliation of life's contradictions. The process not only enhances acceptance (decreasing denial), it also has been found to reduce anxiety about death. This outcome is attributed to the greater meaning achieved through review of one's life and the sense of a legacy developed in the process. Perhaps a person can feel that he or she will still belong to others after death. As Robert Anderson (1970) said, "Death ends a life, but it does not end a relationship."

Georgemiller and Maloney (1984) found that seniors who participated in life review workshops, similar to guided autobiography, were better able to adapt to or handle their own reactions to the possibilities of their own deaths and increased their reminiscing about their lives after the workshop. They noted dramatic, positive outcomes for some participants, as in the case of a woman who was able to resolve much of the resentment and hostility she had been harboring for years against her deceased husband.

Thus, many benefits can be derived from guided autobiography for older adults and others. You as a group leader can help older adults reconcile their pasts and develop increased self-esteem, competence, and a sense of fulfillment. Put simply, members of your guided autobiography group will leave the experience more content with themselves, with their lives, and with their friendships.

Chapter 2

Leading a Guided Autobiography Group

I N GUIDED AUTOBIOGRAPHY, group members are brought together to write and share brief autobiographical life stories of their lives based on assigned themes. The group generally meets ten times for about two hours each time, during which members share nine autobiographical life accounts. Supplemental, optional tasks (as described here and in Chapter 6) can also be used by the group leader to promote understanding of key life issues, to stimulate creativity, and to encourage the development of friendships in the group.

Initiating and leading a guided autobiography group involves the following steps, which form the core discussion of this chapter:

1. Choosing an organization, adult education center, care facility, or residential setting in which the guided autobiography experience will be offered, and designing the process to fit older adults in that facility.
2. Developing materials that (a) describe the guided autobiography process (it is recommended that you adapt the description provided in the first section of Chapter 1 for this purpose), (b) define the goals for the group, (c) discuss group norms, and (d) make it clear that guided autobiography is not, in itself, a form of therapy. This last statement should suggest that those seeking therapy contact a professional therapist.
3. Working with the staff to enlist their cooperation and promote the guided autobiography process to residents or clientele.
4. If possible, speaking with potential group members in person or

over the telephone to repeat and clarify the information provided in the written materials.

5. Leading the group process.
6. Providing support for group members and feedback to staff or family, as applicable.

The Guided Autobiography Process

A person can examine his or her life from a variety of viewpoints—by recalling events as they happened chronologically in time, by focusing on specific events, or by using a major theme, for example, the road taken to achieve success in a career or the events leading to religious revelation. We believe that autobiography is most fruitful for older adults when done as part of a guided process that directs attention to major life themes and when shared in a group. Guided autobiography is based on the conviction that certain themes elicit the most powerful memories and are then most relevant to the issues and needs of older adults. The individual is thus "guided" to make the search of personal history effective and efficient.

An analogy can be drawn to the effectiveness of the old fisherman who always seems to catch fish when others fail. Is it just luck? Obviously not; he has been fishing successfully for many years while others, with good equipment and the right bait, come back empty handed. Yet, when asked to explain his strategy, he says simply, "I know where the fish are."

Many years of experience in conducting guided autobiography groups have resulted in the development of the life themes and sensitizing questions that have proven to be significant guides and stimuli to enhance recall for older adults. One good fishing spot for significant autobiographical material is obviously one's family history. Others include the history of our health and body image, how we got into our life's work, our experiences with loss, our loves and hates. Such themes have been found to elicit rich memories and strong feelings and generally motivate vivid recollections of experience. They often suggest the threads that bind the life story. In Chapters 4 and 5, these themes are described further, and sensitizing questions are presented for each.

Additional themes may be added or substituted depending on the nature and purpose of the group you design. This would be particularly appropriate for groups brought together on the basis of similar histories or current life crises. A list of some sample topics that might be added for such groups is as follows:

Type of Group	Special Topic
Veterans	Impact of being in battle on subsequent re-integration into society
Ethnic minorities or members of special-interest groups	History of political involvement or role of social change in personal development
Members of religious organization	History of spirituality
Upcoming retirees	History of productivity and activities outside the work force
Recovering addicts	Impact of substance abuse on the self and others
Athletes	History of "big games"
Teachers	Students or classes that helped the teacher improve or "grow up" as a teacher
Physicians or lawyers	Cases that will not be forgotten

Since sharing life stories at the group meetings stimulates further recall and interaction, written stories should be restricted to about two pages each to allow enough time for each member to read his or her statement and to allow the opportunity for group feedback. Use the two-page limit as a device to get the participants to focus on key elements of their life stories. Group members may be instructed that this length is a starting point, from which they may choose to expand their autobiography after the group meetings are complete. Sometimes participants may write many pages on a particular theme that stimulates their recall, and they should not feel guilty about it. In the group they should read only two pages since the group process will break down if all the material is presented. The long-winded speaker or the writer who is carried away presents a management problem for the leader of the group, one that is handled with a sense of common purpose and tact (see Chapter 7).

Leadership for a Guided Autobiography Group

The first and most important element in starting a guided autobiography group is a potential leader who has the idea of setting up a group. This idea may grow out of a desire to achieve or impart personal benefits, such as those outlined in the preceding chapter, or may result because it is that person's job to develop such activities. Regardless, the primary impetus is the person who decides to form and conduct the guided autobiography group.

The heart of the group is the leader. You as the leader create the group, maintain its stamina and momentum, and fill a unique role as an intermediary, not only among group members but also between a person and the life story that he or she is retelling.

You set the goals for the group, select its members, and determine much of the group's future identity. According to your purposes, you might choose to bring together new residents in a nursing home, retired physicians, recent widows, or persons with many other common links. Your choice will influence the tone of the group meetings and guide the focus of the writing assignments.

Setting Goals for Group Leaders

You do not have to be a health care professional or therapist to conduct a guided autobiography group. You do have to be a caring, interested person who would like to offer older adults an opportunity to reap as many personal benefits as possible from reviewing their life stories and sharing them with others. The personal attributes of a successful group leader are motivation, warmth, the ability to listen, and the ability to communicate effectively.

It is highly advantageous that leaders participate in guided autobiography before conducting a group. In many settings, however, this is not possible, since they may be the first to introduce the idea. In these cases, an informal group—possibly composed of future group leaders, family, or friends—may be formed in which the leader would participate as a member. An alternative is for the leader to write the autobiographical statements during his or her first experience as a group leader, but not share them in the group.

Nonprofessionals should keep in mind that they are offering an opportunity for older adults to explore their histories and begin to integrate their life stories. They are not offering group psychotherapy and should not probe into the feelings and emotions of group members beyond those that emerge naturally and are shared easily. Group leaders must also protect their members by guarding against such probing by other group members.

Remember also that older people are not as emotionally frail as might be indicated by many of the myths promoted by popular media in our society. Group leaders should not discourage the expression of emotions that are a natural part of interpersonal sharing. Guided autobiography may bring to the surface many of the emotions of the past: sadness and regret over past losses, the joy of "reliving" happy memories, and grief associated with lost loved ones. Unless a group member is demonstrating signs of depression or is at risk (see Chapter 7 for warning signs), a "hands off" philosophy may be best—allowing emotions to emerge naturally as they do in daily life but not soliciting them.

Set reasonable goals for yourself as group leader. Specific goals decrease your uncertainty and confusion concerning your role in the group process. Your role should be based on your personal expertise and what you are comfortable with. We recommend that the leader's goals be kept simple, to allow the group to develop in the most natural way possible. Specific goals might include:

- To arrive early to each meeting and arrange the furniture as needed before the group members' arrival (see section on seating, this chapter). This will create a welcoming atmosphere and avoid the confusion that might occur if members arrive to find an empty or unprepared room.
- To greet each person individually and by name as he or she arrives.
- To encourage each person to read his or her autobiographical statement. Members should be assured that they can skip sections if they are not comfortable discussing them. Less secure members should know that others have an interest in hearing their life stories. Encouragement by the leader is generally welcomed as a sign of support and acceptance.
- To encourage each member to interact with another member at least once during each meeting. This is important for group cohesion and can be accomplished simply by noting similarities among members or asking members to share related experiences.
- To promote group interaction and bonding among members. This is accomplished when a leader allows group members to interact independently. As long as the group rules of acceptance and patience are met, it is not necessary for group leaders to impose order on the interactions following each life story. Group leaders should ensure that no member is interrupted during the reading of his or her life story and should monitor the equal distribution of time

among members. Beyond that, wherever possible, sit back and enjoy the natural course of the interaction in the group.
- To be sincere.
- To never ask any questions you, yourself, would not want to answer and never pressure members to explore topics with which they are not comfortable.
- To be a trusted confidant and to promote confidentiality.
- To listen attentively and acknowledge what is being said. A simple nod of the head, a pass of the tissue when someone is on the verge of tears, or a statement that summarizes an autobiographical life story encourages sharing and emotional security in the group. After a life story is read, leaders may paraphrase some aspect of the story or draw similarities among group members. This lets each member know that he or she is being heard and understood. These concepts are demonstrated in the following example:

Group Member: I guess my early life was fairly sheltered. I did not have to make many decisions. Now that I'm a widow, it's all up to me.

Leader: So the death of your husband put you in the driver's seat. [paraphrases content] That must be exciting, but a bit confusing and intimidating too. [acknowledges emotional content] Emily told a similar story yesterday. How did you adjust, Emily? [acknowledges that Emily, too, has been heard, and promotes interaction]

Co-leading Groups

Particularly for new leaders, or when group size is too large to be manageable by one person (more than six to eight members), co-leadership may be a positive approach to guiding autobiography groups. One should choose a co-leader carefully and discuss fully the division of roles and coordination of leadership *before the first meeting*. Each co-leader's expectations should be addressed and clarified. Also, personal styles should be discussed and strategies should be planned for dealing with interpersonal differences. In cases where group management styles or opinions conflict, negotiations should occur *outside and separate from the group*.

Power struggles can emerge because of a lack of clarity about roles and responsibilities. Problems that emerge, such as frequent refusal by a member to comply with group rules (for example, showing up without assignments) or disagreements among members, should be discussed separately by co-leaders and later brought to the individual or the group. In this way, the co-leaders can present a united front, which is important to maintaining a sense of security among group members. A list of possible role-division strategies that have been successful in co-leading guided autobiography groups is as follows:

Strategy 1

Leader 1

Moderates group discussions of all themes and written life stories

Leader 2

Monitors time limits and group reactions and looks for warning signs of distress or depression among members (see Chapter 7)

Strategy 2

Leader 1

Presents theme assignments and moderates discussion of theme assignments in advance of writing

Leader 2

Moderates reading of life stories on the theme for the day and group discussion of the member's written life stories

Strategy 3

Leader 1

Leads group meetings

Leader 2

Makes logistical arrangements and coordinates communication with group members as needed outside the group

Selecting and Training Other Leaders

If there is an unexpected overenrollment of one group or if the leader wishes to extend guided autobiography groups beyond his or her own capacity to lead them, it may be necessary and beneficial to develop a network of group leaders. Such a network requires careful selection and training.

The authors have created a number of such networks, including some in the community, among older volunteers, among a group of college alumni, and in a retirement village. It is advantageous to select leaders who have participated as members in your guided autobiography groups. They provide the experience from which training can progress, and they have the motivation to offer this opportunity to others.

You should consider whether potential leaders are suited to the role of moderator. Persons chosen should demonstrate open personalities that encourage acceptance and support. Of special importance is for group leaders to approach guided autobiography with an interest in hearing other peoples' stories and without a desire to monopolize the group with their own interpretations and life experiences. Issues of confidentiality should be discussed at length, and only people who demonstrate an ability and desire to maintain confidentiality should be chosen as group leaders.

Potential group leaders can be helped through the use of information and suggestions in this book, especially this chapter and the sections that focus on the leader's role in developing group cohesion, stimulating creative thinking, and mastering potential problems in the group. Informing your leaders of the benefits and theories that inspired your own desire to conduct guided autobiography groups will motivate them. The chapters that relate to these issues can be read and discussed with the leaders during the training process. This training can be enhanced by anecdotes from your personal experiences in leading guided autobiography.

Group leaders should meet after their first independently led guided autobiography group meeting in order to discuss their experiences, review group goals and group rules, and address any problems that may have occurred or may be anticipated. Such meetings among group leaders should take place periodically, for example, about every three sessions.

Creating the Group

The group leader's influence begins long before the first meeting. Your expertise in selecting and preparing group members will in large part determine the group's success and influence the potential for group cohesion and continuity. In this regard, choose group members who are seriously interested in the process, who will plan to attend all sessions if at all possible, and who agree on a set of group goals and rules.

This is best accomplished through the use of well-written materials that describe the group process and the rules for all members. Such materials might be distributed in advance of the first meeting then reviewed at the first meeting. A good opening for descriptive materials is as follows:

All of us need to believe that our lives have mattered, that we have had a purpose or impact on the world. Guided autobiography can help you to explore what you have accomplished. Doing a guided autobiography can help you to identify life-long strengths that can assist adaptation in your later years; it can provide insight about where you have come from as you face the new crossroads in your life. By completing a guided autobiography, you can create an important legacy for your family.

Guided autobiography combines individual and group experiences with autobiography, including (1) private reflection and the writing of two-page life stories on selected life themes and (2) reading these life stories and sharing thoughts in a group. Sharing life stories with other group members refreshes one's memories of the past and allows individuals to reexperience parts of themselves in the stories of others.

The guided autobiography group will meet (dates, times, place). You will be asked to write and share with the group a series of brief autobiographical life stories based on the following themes: (insert themes you have chosen for the group).

Next, you would include the goals and guidelines for participation. In the following sections, we define appropriate goals for the group and discuss group norms. Once you read these sections, consider carefully which points are applicable to your target audience and extract them for use in the description of the process.

Setting Goals for Group Members

Goals for group members should derive from your own motivation to conduct guided autobiography and from the unique aspects of your specific group. General group goals should be:

- For members to get to know each other
- To share life stories
- To explore similarities and differences among group members
- To share life strategies
- To make each member feel that there is confidentiality and trust in the group
- To encourage the elaboration of each person's life story

Other group goals are derived from the purposes that determine the compilation of a specific group and are a product of the identifying nature of that group. Just some examples might include:

- For members to meet or begin integrating into a new setting (e.g., nursing home life)
- For members to explore life strategies that might be applied to new

demands or life transitions, for example, widowhood, disability, or retirement

- For members to explore how they have arrived at a certain life point, for example, imprisonment for a crime, and to begin exploring new or alternative directions
- For members to begin coming to terms with impending death

These group goals are in addition to the personal goals of the different members. Personal goals may vary and be as different as the group members themselves. They include personal growth, self-understanding, creation of a family legacy, and other potential outcomes described in Chapter 1. Regardless of each member's personal goals, however, all written materials and conversations before the first session should identify the group goals and note their importance to help ensure a spirit of camaraderie and sharing.

The Design of the Group

The nature of the group should be decided by the group leader. Then descriptive materials can be designed, and members can be recruited (either via self-selection or through the assistance of staff) who fit the category selected (such as recent retirees). The leader may want to take into account backgrounds and personality types when combining people into a group. In addition, the leader should note in all written materials and early discussions the importance of maintaining continuity of the group and should request a commitment to completing the process to the degree possible.

For the authors, the prototypic group includes men and women from a wide age range (age 20 to 88) and diverse ethnic backgrounds and careers who have participated as part of a summer course at a major university. Among the environments where this approach has proven to be well suited are:

- Universities and colleges
- Religious institutions
- Community centers
- Counseling facilities
- Community educational facilities

Other groups have consisted of particular cohorts, people of the same generation with a common historical connection. This type of group can provide a unique opportunity for shared memories. In many cases, a common historical context serves as a catalyst for a life story, particularly in times of upheaval, such as the Depression era or the 1960s. Common memories can stimulate further recall and provide the opportunity to view major life influences from the perspective of others. This type of group is particularly suited to the environment of a nursing home or senior center in that it promotes camaraderie and the opportunity for shared reminiscences. The following is a sampling of the kind of cohort groups that might be brought together:

- People who grew up in the Depression
- Veterans of particular wars
- Concentration camp survivors
- People who went to college during the 1960s
- Women who entered the work force in the early feminist period (late 1960s and early 1970s)
- Immigrants from the same historical period
- Regional farmers, for example, those who experienced the Dust Bowl of the early 1930s

Other groups might be brought together by a current purpose, for example, a shared profession or current life crisis. Two such groups in the past have been a group of physicians who practiced in the same geographic area and a group of older adults who recently suffered the loss of an adult child.

Selecting and Recruiting Members

Once the goals and design of the group have been set, it is time to select and recruit members. As group leader, it is important for you to be involved in this process. If possible, it would be beneficial for you to meet or engage in a telephone conversation with each member before acceptance into the group. If this is not possible, you can guide self-selection by including clear statements of criteria and goals in all written materials. Members should be advised to join the group only if they agree with the group goals and will comply with group rules (appropriate rules are discussed below).

Wherever possible, it is advantageous to use the valuable resources and information provided by facility staff and caretakers who can help identify and screen potential group members. They are also an important resource in encouraging members to join a group and in assisting members to ensure consistent and prompt attendance.

Although almost anyone *can* participate, group leaders should consider the effective functioning of the group when choosing members. For example, it would not be beneficial to create a group that is composed of members who differ widely in degree of cognitive disturbance, such as a group that combined well-functioning older adults with the severely demented. Burnside (1984) suggested that the following be excluded from well-functioning groups:

- Disturbed, active, wandering persons
- Patients with psychotic depression
- People who do not participate on their own recognizance, for example, who are coerced by others to attend
- Individuals diagnosed as having bipolar disorder
- Persons who are unable to communicate effectively with other group members because of a physical or cognitive disability
- Hypochondriacal persons

To this list might be added persons with paranoid personality disorders and persons suffering from delusional states.

The goal of guided autobiography is to involve the essentially normal, adapting person. It is not oriented toward use with such persons as Burnside lists. An appropriate selection is fairly simple to achieve in institutional settings, where staff can help you to choose among potential group members. The emphasis on selection of members in the community, however, heavily rests on self-selection, which is why we stress the importance of including a statement in all literature that this is not therapy for specific problems. It is not advised that psychological screening be attempted in any formal way, since this will confuse potential members by placing a therapylike emphasis on entrance into the group.

There may be an occasional disturbed person who might enter a group, but he or she will exit quickly when needs are not being served. If an inappropriate member stays in the group, you can use the techniques described in Chapter 7 on managing the problem group member.

In an institutional setting, potential members should be screened for noticeable cognitive disability, for example, the ability to concentrate and stick to a theme, the ability to listen, or the ability to reason. Although successful groups have been conducted with the cognitively impaired, it is suggested that noticeable differences in cognitive level not be mixed within a given group.

Finally, if a potential member indicates that therapy is desired, such a person should be referred to an expert medical health care provider or agency.

Fostering Group Participation

Particularly with older adults, new members may be shy or anxiously resistant to participating in group discussions. Simple strategies can promote participation and enhance the group experience. For example, coffee, tea, and snacks have been found to increase attendance at most group meetings. After these are brought first by the group leader, the group may wish to rotate the responsibility for bringing snacks. This enhances commitment to the group and is a way of sharing one's self with others. It can be elaborated by each member bringing a dish that is part of his or her heritage. Also, it is a method for preventing member attrition; members are brought back into the group when it is their turn to bring a snack.

In addition to the enticement of snacks, opportunities to show family photographs or to listen to music from one's past can be created and integrated as ways to attract and sustain participation. This can also have positive effects for recall of events and persons. Distant memories can be brought to mind by old photographs (e.g., wedding pictures) and the emotions reexperienced.

During the time span of the guided autobiography group meetings, the leader may be called upon to act as a gatekeeper, to minimize absenteeism and member attrition. It may be necessary to intervene if a member frequently arrives late, is absent, or does not prepare a written statement to share with the group. If absent, a member should be asked to prepare the written autobiographical statement for the meeting missed and should be encouraged to briefly share this statement with other group members upon his or her return. This is important since the guided autobiography process is a cumulative one that provides a sense of completion for all members. Keeping the person in tempo with the group process through regular attendance is important.

Group Culture and Rules

You as the group leader take initiative in creating a subculture for the group, establishing the rules that govern its conduct and helping to guide the development of relationships among members. You should describe and, most importantly, *model* the "game rules" that govern group interactions, particularly setting a nonjudgmental atmosphere of acceptance and support. (How this is accomplished is discussed at length in Chapter 3.) What is important here is that group rules are established relatively early in the life of a group and are later difficult to change. Therefore, in advance of the first meeting, it is essential for you to consider carefully what rules, or patterns of behavior, should be developed in the group and to make these rules clear to potential group members before they join the group.

Some group rules that are particularly beneficial to guided autobiography are:

- Willingness to share your life story with others
- Commitment to attend all meetings, if at all possible
- Willingness to complete and share all writing assignments
- Being an attentive listener when others are sharing
- Striving to be supportive of others and accepting of individual differences
- Avoiding judgmental statements about the choices other members have made or about their feelings, beliefs, or opinions
- Confidentiality
- Avoiding comparisons that imply judgments of "right" and "wrong," "better" and "worse," or "success" and "failure"

At the first meeting of the group, these rules should again be discussed to ensure clarity and understanding. During the meetings, the leader should model the standards that have been agreed upon by the group and should monitor and intervene when necessary to maintain adequate compliance and the security of all group members.

In addition to acceptance and support, an effort should be made by all members to listen to each other. Participants may become impatient with a slow speaker, or, in an effort to make sure they have a chance to speak and be listened to, may attempt to rush the discussion of other members' stories. The best way to avoid such problems is to model good listening behavior and to set reasonable and clear limits on time so that each member is guaranteed an opportunity to speak and be heard. You are responsible for monitoring time and directing the group's focus. Older adults, particularly those who are experiencing social isolation or the need to adjust to age-related declines, require time to sort through their memories and emotions. We recommend that the size of such groups be kept small—about six members.

Developing Group Cohesion

Group members are often strangers before the first meeting, so you serve as a "home base" from which relationships with others in the group can be explored, and trust and acceptance developed.

Particularly in working with older adults, you may find that during the first session group members will tend to speak only to you. As the group leader, you play an important role in connecting the members to each other, stimulating interaction, trust, and social bonding. You can achieve this by noting similarities among group members to facilitate their interaction. In the following example, a group leader, Judy, uses a subtle technique to join two men who, by the third meeting, had yet to interact much with other members in the group.

> John (Member): I first became interested in plants when I spent the summer of seventh grade on my grandfather's farm. I've loved gardening ever since. It's what I miss most living here.
>
> Judy (Leader): So, you had to leave your garden behind when you moved here. You must feel a lot like Alan felt when he was unable to bring along his tools—later he worked it out with the activities director by donating them to the craft room. Now you do some odd jobs around the home, don't you Alan? Maybe you could tell John who he might speak to in order to arrange something similar.

Remember, however, that the process may be slow, particularly with older adults who have left old friends and are facing new demands. They may be experiencing crises in maintaining a sense of self-worth and may be slow to develop feelings of trust with other group members. Also, they may have a strong, competing desire to be specially recognized by the group leader. You should try to make all members feel that they are equally important to the group by focusing group members' attention on their own capacities to support and validate each other.

The Logistics of Meetings

A successful group experience in guided autobiography is the result of the development of rules that encourage the acceptance and participation of all members. It is also the result of planned leadership and attention to details. In the following sections we discuss more detailed recommendations regarding group design, content, and logistical arrangements.

Times and Length

The guided autobiography group usually meets ten times; this represents one meeting for each life-story theme plus an introductory meeting. The process can be completed in an intensive experience of meeting every day for two weeks (exclusive of weekends), it can be extended over ten weeks, meeting once a week, or it can combine elements of these schedules. Particularly in nursing homes and senior centers, group members may decide to continue meeting after the structured process is complete.

Frequently, older adults prefer to meet early in the day; they generally do not want to meet in the evenings, particularly if it would require travelling away from their homes. In institutional settings, it is also important to choose a time that is consistent with the needs of the staff. Any disruption of the routine should be avoided, and one must keep in mind the importance of staff compliance in ensuring that members are ready and able to attend the meetings.

Each group meeting should be scheduled for a minimum of two hours since it must include both the sensitizing discussion and the exchange of autobiographical statements. The individual reading time is typically fifteen to twenty minutes. More than two hours will be needed if the group number increases beyond five or six or if the process is part of a course that includes discussion of issues of human development. Longer sessions also have to include restroom and, often, coffee breaks, resulting in three-hour sessions.

The First Meeting

At the first meeting, you as the leader should ask all members to introduce themselves and make one or two statements about why they are interested in autobiography and something about their current lives. You should introduce yourself and ask leading questions, such as:

Where do you live?
Where did you grow up?
Whom do you live with?
What was or is your career?

This might be followed with some discussion about why members decided to engage in guided autobiography. In this regard, you might share some ideas about the potential outcomes of the technique and stimulate members to expand their views.

Next, the ground rules should be explained and discussed with the group. In your opening statements, you should include the following points:

1. Each member should be aware of meeting dates, times, and length.
2. Each member will bring a two-page life story on a specific topic to each meeting. Each person will read aloud his or her two pages. It is important to emphasize the two-page length of each life story and to comment about the importance of each member having an opportunity to read. You might note that many participants go on to expand the writing of their autobiographies after the group process has ended.
3. A one-page list of sensitizing questions on each theme will be distributed and discussed before each meeting (see Chapter 5). These questions are meant to stimulate thinking and to guide *but not to structure or limit one's thinking*. This last point should be reinforced at each session.
4. Interaction in the group is promoted in a nonjudgmental atmosphere of acceptance and support. Here, you might briefly describe and discuss the developmental exchange (see Chapter 3) and focus attention on the importance of creating an environment where every member feels welcome and able to share his or her life stories. The group rules described earlier in this chapter should be agreed upon by all members.

The group might also be encouraged to decide on policies regarding missed meetings. Such policies are important to ensure a smooth road for the developmental exchange (see Chapter 3). It is recommended that all members plan to attend every meeting. It is not recommended that a member be part of a group if he or she will miss more than two of the ten sessions.

The life story based on the theme of Branching Points (see Chapter 5) should be the first assignment. It should be handed out and discussed at the first meeting, then two pages on the topic should be written by each member and read at the second meeting.

The Format of the Meeting

At each meeting, approximately twenty minutes to a half hour should be devoted to discussion of the sensitizing questions that will guide the following meeting's life story. You should pass out and read aloud a description of the topic and a sampling of the sensitizing questions (see Chapter 5). In doing so, you might share some of your own thoughts and experiences related to the topic as a way to initiate group discussion. In addition, you might ask the group some questions derived from the sensitizing material. Discussion of the topic at this point should be kept brief and moderated by you, as group leader. The goal is to stimulate thinking and expand members' perspectives regarding how a topic might be approached. As necessary, members should be made aware of this goal and of their opportunity to write about the topic and share their experiences at the next meeting. (A discussion of the importance of sensitization in the autobiography process is presented in Chapter 4.)

Approximately one-and-a-half hours should be devoted to the reading of that day's life stories, allowing about fifteen minutes for each (usually, ten to fifteen minutes of reading and five minutes of group interaction). The leader should moderate this interaction to ensure that the group remains nonjudgmental and that each member has a turn of approximately equal length.

The Size of the Group

The number of people in a group is the decision of the group leader. The smaller the group, however, the more interaction occurs. Because of the time needed to read and comment on each member's life story, the most effective groups consist of about five to eight members. A number of groups are often conducted simultaneously as space and number of leaders permit. The authors often have six groups meeting at the same time.

Too many members will result in a group that is not manageable. People may be cut short or not have an opportunity to read their life story or provide insight into the life story of others. Too few members may result in a group that does not have enough content, limiting the potential for similarities and contrasts to be drawn. Most importantly, too few members at the beginning can result in the breaking apart of the group should one or two members become ill, travel, or choose to leave.

It is not recommended that new members be added after the second session, since this will disrupt the natural progression of sharing in the group and the formation of a cohesive group. Should a new member be added, he or she should be asked to complete the previous life stories before entry into the group. The new member should summarize the content of these life stories at the first meeting attended.

Settings

The setting for the guided autobiography group meetings can vary widely and is dependent on group size, the number of groups being conducted simultaneously, and the physical needs of participants (e.g., wheelchair access). Ideally, the groups should meet in separate rooms, quiet and free from distractions, that will provide the privacy necessary for personal disclosure.

Drawing on a list developed by Burnside (1984), settings might include:

Community centers
Schools
Hospitals
Board-and-care and nursing homes
Mental health facilities
Churches or synagogues
Private residences
Business organizations
Prisons
Rehabilitation centers
Outpatient facilities
Recreation and park areas
Retirement communities
Senior centers
Veterans Administration hospitals and centers
Volunteer centers

Seating Arrangements

In conducting the guided autobiography group, seating arrangements can be made around a table or by simply putting chairs in a circle. Such arrangements should allow for close proximity of group members and for each member to be able to easily look at and speak to every other member. A table has the advantage of providing a place to write and set down a cup of coffee or snack.

An important aspect of group leadership and co-leadership is the location of group leaders. Seating arrangements should be designed consistent with the roles agreed upon and with the goal of facilitating group interaction and listening. It is important to keep in mind that some older adults experience age-related hearing losses, so seating should be arranged such that group members are close to each other. If possible, all group members should be in nearly equal proximity to a leader and should experience no visual obstructions in speaking with a leader. Arrangements should be made as necessary for wheelchair access and positioning of wheelchair-bound participants in the natural constellation of the group.

Wherever possible, seating should be arranged in a circle, with co-leaders sitting opposite each other. Squares are difficult since they result in unequal visual access. People tend not to interact with those they can not see and may become impatient with listening if they feel they are not part of the direct audience. Rectangular or octagonal arrangements result in unequal weighing of proximity, but they can be used if co-leaders sit diagonally to afford each group member with a feeling of equal access.

Costs and Expenses

It is difficult for us to estimate the costs for you to conduct a guided autobiography group, since much relies on the setting you choose and the institutional support received. Here we will attempt to address the potential costs that must be considered and some ways to manage these costs. First, we will discuss four methods by which costs for these groups are traditionally met.

1. Many group leaders initiate guided autobiography as part of their existing jobs. Thus, costs may be subsumed under existing salaries and program/project budgets.
2. In other cases, support may come from the facilities in which guided autobiography is being offered, either through visiting instructorships or existing funding for programs and services, with the group leader acting as a consultant to the facility.
3. A traditional method for covering costs is through revenues generated by charging participants for enrollment. This frequently results in a self-selection process whereby only those older adults who can afford to participate become group members. Given the limited, fixed incomes of many seniors, amounts charged are usually nominal to avoid excluding large numbers. Still, this model has been used successfully in facilities offering continuing education, in which most participants have achieved high educational levels and adequate financial status. Charges for participation in the guided autobiography groups in different areas and at differ-

ent kinds of facilities range from \$100 to \$750 for a ten-session group process.

4. The fourth model is an informal one, whereby a community of interested persons support the conduct of the group in which they participate, by opening their homes for use or by providing services. This is often successful in retirement communities.

Expenses to be considered in designing a group include the following:

Setting. The largest potential cost is related to the setting in which the guided autobiography group is to be conducted. If this is an entrepreneurial endeavor, space in a community facility may have to be rented. Often, in other settings—such as community colleges, churches and synagogues, nursing homes, older-adult activity centers—the cost for space will be covered by the facility in exchange for the service or for a percentage of enrollment charges (if applicable). In the community, there is also the opportunity to initiate groups in more informal settings. One group leader, for example, has started a series of groups in a retirement community. In this case, members can rotate the use of their homes for meetings.

Personnel. Another primary cost is for personnel, including group leaders and secretarial support to publicize the opportunity to participate and to enroll participants.

Written materials. Promotional materials, including the information on group goals and rules described earlier in this chapter, will have to be designed, printed or copied, and distributed. Depending on the setting chosen and whether (and how much) participants will be charged, these may range from fairly slick promotional brochures to photocopies of typed information. The statements of themes and sensitizing questions (see Chapter 5) also should be reproduced and distributed to all group members, sequentially over the course of the meetings.

"Coffee breaks." In many cases you may want to offer beverages and snacks at meetings. Arrangements can be made among group members to share the responsibility for snacks; beverages are commonly provided by the group leader. Associated costs should be considered in estimating expenses.

Chapter **3**

The Healing Power of the Group

O NCE YOU have planned the guided autobiography group, made the logistical arrangements, and selected and recruited members, it is time to face the crowd. In Chapter 2, we discussed the content and structure of the first meeting. In this chapter, we will discuss the theoretical bases for leading the guided autobiography process in the context of a group experience. Successful techniques will be described and illustrated. Next, we will review the potential benefits of group experiences for older adults and the importance of coupling this with personal reflection and writing. Although, overall, the group process is of great benefit to individuals, there are potential problems that may arise from time to time. The current chapter focuses on the benefits; Chapter 7 presents techniques for managing potential concerns.

Developmental Exchange

A key feature of guided autobiography is the *developmental exchange,* the mutual sharing among members of who they are and where they come from, their personally important historical and emotional events. As each group member reads his or her thematic life story in the small group, the exchange of one's past with other persons reinforces and sustains the motivation to review one's life. This also provides the context for the development of new friendships and greater self-esteem. In addition, we believe that the confidence and trust built through a small group experience enhances both recall and the ease of translating experience to the written page.

Grotjahn (1989) makes the point that the "assignment for the elderly is the integration of past-life experiences into final identity formation"

(p. 110) and suggests this is best done in a group. Group meetings of seniors are coming to be viewed as important not only in consolidating a sense of identity but also in providing relief from feelings of neglect and isolation from life. Yalom (1975) developed twelve general categories of curative factors derived from the group process in therapy:

1. Altruism
2. Group cohesiveness
3. Universality
4. Interpersonal learning: "input"
5. Intrapersonal learning: "output"
6. Guidance
7. Catharsis
8. Identification
9. Family reenactment
10. Insight
11. Instillation of hope
12. Existential enlightenment (meaning)

Although guided autobiography is not designed to be therapy per se, such therapeutic gains can also result from the technique. They are optimized when guided autobiography is conducted in a group.

Sharing in the Group

People who are involved in an incremental developmental exchange during guided autobiography move from tentatively and guardedly alluding to important features of their lives toward an increasingly open sharing of significant personal information. In the process, people implicitly take into account the affective importance of shared information. They trade personal information equivalent in its affective value, though not necessarily similar in content. As time together increases and more of each life is shared, the developmental exchange leads to an increased willingness toward self-disclosure. Friendships and affective bonds are built among group members as mutual respect and trust grow. Increased confidence and trust among group members results not only in a greater willingness to share but also in a greater courage to explore. An example of how a developmental exchange might work, as members trade increasing amounts of personal information, is as follows:

Sara tells John she was born on the eastern seaboard.

John tells Sara his family were fishermen.

Sara tells John her father did not work due to a disability, and so she had to help support the family as a teenager.

John tells Sara that he was once out of work, and so he could relate to what her father must have felt when he was unable to provide for his family. And he goes on to describe a feeling of disempowerment as a result of his recent retirement.

Sara tells John of her own sense of failure when she got her divorce.

John and Sara begin to discuss and, in discussing, evaluate how they derive their feelings of self-worth.

As the example illustrates, the developmental exchange goes much like a poker game in which each player increases the ante of information and feelings on his or her turn. If a player does not want to proceed further, the last player's ante is simply met or the player passes. By meeting the ante, the player can remain part of the group but maintain the investment at a plateau. If the player chooses instead to drop out, the exchange is halted, perhaps to be resumed at a later date when confidence returns.

Promoting the Developmental Exchange

In a group consisting of complete strangers or people who have met only briefly, there is an initial reluctance to share thoughts and feelings. Early in the group process, an easy-to-write theme may be difficult to read. Without the group leader, the developmental exchange may be delayed or arrested or may sustain itself at a superficial level. As a group leader, you can promote this exchange through the use of three primary strategies:

Strategy 1: Linking group members who have discussed similar stories or who may have pertinent suggestions. This strategy was introduced earlier and can be used in many group experiences. All that is required is good listening skills and the ability to draw connections between personal experiences. When you demonstrate both qualities, you (1) provide members with a feeling of confidence that they have something interesting and important to add, (2) present the message that you, as the resident authority, welcome interaction among members, and (3) draw attention to the opportunity for and appropriateness of such interaction. The approach can be both simple and soft, as demonstrated in the following example:

> At the end of his life-story essay on the history of his career and life's work, John discloses that his retirement has left him feeling useless and that he does not know what to do with his time. His disclosure is met with empty stares from the other group members who have yet to disclose such personal information.
>
> Leader: It sounds as though you are experiencing a transition that will require some adjustment. This is not unlike Martha's story about her need to find work after all her children were grown and had left home.
>
> Once the connection has been pointed out, Martha and others who have experienced similar role losses may begin to share some of their own feelings.

Strategy 2: Sharing your own thoughts or questions about what has just been said. At times, particularly in working with older adults, it is important to demonstrate that you not only are hearing what they have to say but are genuinely interested in their life stories. This can promote further disclosure by the person already speaking or may prompt others to express similar thoughts, experiences, or feelings. The developmental exchange is catalyzed by the value you apply to it through your interest.

> In his life story essay on "Major Branching Points," Sam tells the group about layoffs in his father's factory, which led to his decision to quit college during the Depression. As his story ends, the group looks to the leader with unspoken questions about what will happen next.
>
> Leader: So many of you come from different backgrounds, I wonder what your experiences were during the Depression. Sam, what was it like on the farm?

In this example, the leader expresses a personal interest in the topic and promotes an exchange of stories surrounding it. Such an approach stimulates memories and motivates participants. In short, it models an atmosphere of mutual respect and enjoyment.

Strategy 3: The subtle use of self-disclosure. We recommend that you as the group leader facilitate interactions *between and among group members* as a primary role. This involves careful monitoring of your own involvement in the group process of sharing life stories. In some cases, you may choose also to participate to some extent as a member of the group. In general, however, this is not recommended. When you write or share personal autobiographical statements, there may be competition for your role as moderator, and you may inhibit exchanges and cause a feeling of inequality among other members.

It is also important, however, for members to feel that the leader is an impartial ally and to experience a sense of reciprocity. To accomplish this and to promote the developmental exchange, group leaders can engage in the occasional subtle use of self-disclosure.

This strategy is employed when the group leader interjects a brief personal vignette or shares an emotion. It is best used when it is designed to highlight similarities among human experiences or universalities in human emotions. This insertion of an item by the leader is particularly important in situations where a member may feel alone or ostracized by the group. It can be an effective antidote in instances when the developmental exchange moves too quickly, when rules are breached, or when privacy is invaded. The next example recounts an instance in which a group leader skillfully deflected an unfair judgment through the use of personal disclosure:

> Alan (in closing his life story on the theme of bereavement): I have not attended any family gatherings since my wife's death. I just can't seem to do it.
>
> Mary: That seems abnormal to me. I would think you would want to be around your family *more.*
>
> Leader: I don't know. Alan's feelings make sense to me. I lost a grandchild once and, for a while, I didn't want to go anywhere if I thought there would be babies around. Sometimes it's hard to be with the people that remind you most of a loved one just after their death.
>
> The next day, this leader opened the group with the following statement: "It's our third meeting and at this point I usually take the opportunity to review some of our game rules. . . ." She went on to briefly remind the members of all the rules to which they had agreed, but she lingered just a bit longer on the importance of being nonjudgmental.

Mutual Acceptance and Support

Paradoxically, what may have been difficult to write is sometimes easily expressed in the group context. This is particularly true as it relates to the impact of group acceptance and support on a person's willingness to "dig deeper." New associations may arise from the group discussion, as the facts and feelings take on a living quality for both readers and listeners. Other people's experiences become reminders of feelings and events that we have set aside and thought we had forgotten.

In addition, the distribution of attention among group members has the effect of reducing pressure on any one person and providing support in dealing with painful memories. One role of the group is to assist other members who become "stuck" at some painful point in the past, providing the stimulus to move on to new territory.

As group leader, you play an important part in this process. When you perceive a noticeable shift in attitude on the part of a member or become conscious of nonverbal behavior that indicates that the member is uncomfortable discussing a topic, you can help the member by changing the subject or moving on to a new topic. A vital resource in such instances is the use of the clock. Group members will soon become used to and, indeed, rely on your role as timekeeper. Even if not precise, this role can be employed to move the group's focus away from a person who is usurping the group's attention or is experiencing difficulty, to give a person time to regroup and reenter group interactions once he or she is on more secure emotional ground. As a group matures, such deflection is rarely called for.

Interpersonal Relations

Many facets of the interpersonal relationships developed in the group contribute to the experience, insight, and confidence gained by participating in guided autobiography. In this section, we will highlight aspects of the group process that are particularly constructive.

Tears

It is okay for group members occasionally to become upset and cry. If the person appears reasonably comfortable sharing his or her emotions and if the other group members are not significantly disturbed by the emotional display, tears can often act as a catalyst to further bonding. By creating an atmosphere where the trials and hardships of life can be shared, the group can affirm the person's ability to proceed beyond a troubling event and aid in the development of greater confidence and self-worth. You can assist in this process by demonstrating your own comfort with, and acceptance of, the emotion being displayed.

We have often seen tears unite group members in a way that no other occurrence in the group seems to foster. Tears are a demonstration of a need to express feelings of intense sadness or joy but are also a demonstration of trust and humanity. Another person's tears expose the vulnerabilities in all of us and frequently trigger the desire to protect and support the other person. They represent high "stakes" in the developmental exchange and are usually met with reciprocal trust and an increased willingness to share highly personal recollections and emotions.

We are always impressed with the impact of a group leader's saying, "Sometimes people cry during group meetings. In fact, many people do at least once." This information frees the group. Older adults, like everyone else, sometimes need permission before they are willing or able to risk interaction on a highly emotional plane. The best advice we can offer is bring a box of tissues, and do not take the occurrence of tears too seriously. It is not a sign something has gone wrong. It is a sign something is going right.

Once tears are being shed, carefully observe the emotional level. You must decide when it is time to move on. This can be based on a decision that the next person's time has come, particularly if you begin to note impatience on the part of other members or increasing discomfort or agitation among the group. Because this is not therapy, it is important to make sure that an occasionally strong emotional display does not spiral into feelings of despair. (See also Chapter 7 for warning signals indicating that a person should be referred to professional assistance.)

Often you can bring a person to emotional closure effectively and sensitively through the use of nonverbal behavior. A smile, quick hug, pat on the hand, or the passing of a box of tissues breaks the mood, sends a message of empathetic support, and lets a person know it is time to move along. A simple statement acknowledging the emotion can be carefully followed by words that direct attention to the next person and tell that person to read his or her life story.

Support and Personal Growth

Not all life experiences are negative. There are many high moments in life to recall. Past successes and good relationships can easily be overlooked. They are often brought to mind by the recollections of others in the group. The leader can point out that the ups as well as the downs are important in clarifying our views of our past. More realistic views are likely to emerge as a result of group feedback, which gives participants a sense of permission and acceptance to talk about successes and failures.

The "Oh" Phenomenon

One aspect of the role of support in personal growth might best be termed the *"Oh" phenomenon*. This is seen when a person comes to guided autobiography with what he or she perceives as a "dark secret," some act or feeling from the past that makes one feel separate and unacceptable. Revelation of this secret in the group is often met with little surprise or judgment. In fact, it is often met with similar revelations or simple acceptance. In essence, the other group members say, "Oh, that's nothing."

Such an experience can be extremely freeing. A person may leave the group that day with the feeling that a weight has been lifted, as in the following example:

> Ann grew up in a household that stressed socially "correct" behaviors and how such behaviors determine proper fit and success in life roles. She viewed her own role as that of "mother" and judged her success by the degree to which *all* her behaviors fitted with her interpretation of that role. Divergence from those behaviors was a sign of failure.
>
> Ann had a "dark secret," which she believed was a sure sign of such failure. Early in her marriage she had had a brief affair, during a weekend visit with a friend in another city. Despite her subsequent fidelity and dedication to her husband and now adult children, Ann was sure that revelation of her secret would make her unacceptable.
>
> During Ann's experience in guided autobiography, the topic of infidelity emerged in Jerry's, another member's, life-story essay on the theme of family. Ann was surprised to discover how freely Jerry discussed his sexual history and the impact of an affair on his still-intact marriage. She was equally surprised to note the group leader's acceptance of this information and its lack of impact on his treatment of Jerry in the group.
>
> The next day, she was even more surprised to find herself talking of her own affair and to discover that the group leader and the others did not comprehend the value she placed on it in defining her success as a mother. This experience made her rethink her assessment of her successes and failures. Set in the con-

text of an entire life span, this one episode was put into a new and more realistic perspective.

Clearly, in your role as leader you are important in promoting such acceptance. Members may look to you for cues or guidance about how to respond. Your nonverbal behaviors may provide the cues that steer interactions and determine whether other members will be willing to share similar information. In all cases, you must model and enforce the rule of being nonjudgmental.

Similarity and Uniqueness in Life Histories

The group experience provides the opportunity for people to see themselves reflected in the stories of others. In a sense, each member of the group holds up a mirror in which others can see themselves from a new angle. Each participant is enriched by the opportunity to see similarities in experience and to emerge with confidence in the universality of people. Contrasts develop and the range of individual differences becomes apparent, helping to clarify the person's sense of distinct identity.

Similarities of experience among group members can help a participant feel accepted and, equally important, acceptable. The experience of Ann demonstrates this outcome. This acceptance is key to our mental well-being and can provide a solid base of departure for further exploration into the self and for future action.

Acceptance plays an even more important role in the case of contrasts. In achieving a sense that one is unique and yet still welcome, a participant can gain increased security in his or her own abilities and enhanced self-worth.

Anonymity and Confidentiality

Many people who participate in guided autobiography choose to do so in a group of people with whom they have no other connections. This "anonymity" provides a protected sphere in which to explore the self; their friends do not have to know everything. Revelations are made with greater freedom since the "cost" is limited if the revelations are viewed negatively. In a sense, one is freer to explore the inner world of the self when one's personal outer world is not watching or hanging on to every word. This perspective was brought to the attention of the authors through an anecdote told by a past participant in guided autobiography:

This participant had recently attended a group reunion in which one member laughed and said, "If I had known I would see you all again, I would have never told you all that I did!"

This member, now over age 70, was for years an esteemed community leader and very active in her church. She had joined in many secret love affairs over the course of her life, but she kept these relationships clandestine because of her role in her church and community. She had disclosed her past to the group only because it had no bearing on her social milieu.

Asked if she wished she had not divulged the information, she said, "Of course not, I trust you now."

Not all persons seek anonymity, and many enjoy sharing their life histories with those they are closest to or with whom they have a common connection. One potential benefit for groups that are brought together randomly is that members can choose to remain somewhat anonymous, keeping the experience separate from other aspects of their life; or members may share all or parts of their autobiographies with others outside the group during or after the series of group sessions. However, they are told not to retell the life events that others in their group relate. This brings us to the important issue of *confidentiality*.

Confidentiality is an important group rule. Without it, there can be no true sense of openness or sharing. It is imperative to model this standard in all your interactions within and outside the group. In this regard, carefully consider references to past group members. You should note that in all examples given in this book, names and identifying information have been changed. Members must be assured that confidentiality will exist even beyond the life of the group.

Issues of confidentiality should be discussed with each member prior to commitment to the group and should be repeated on the first day. Particularly with older adults in institutional settings, privacy is often a serious concern. Care should be taken to maintain confidentiality not only among members, but also with regard to staff of the institution. The degree to which members feel confident that their secrets will remain in the group will determine the degree to which they are willing to explore and share meaningful information.

Humor

Along with the emotional recall of an early mishap or a broken love relationship, there are often humorous recollections that can have a profound effect on feelings of release and relief and that are enjoyable to share with the group. You should stress that in the group, members can share important memories of all tones and colors. This is particularly important as part of your assurance that you are not conducting group therapy. Likewise, it is an important factor in recruiting and maintaining membership, since it plays a primary role in keeping the group experience fun.

Researchers (e.g., Vaillant, 1977) have found that humor promotes the development of ease with the self. That is, the use of humor about the self helps a person accept, or at least understand, who and how he or she is. With humor, vulnerabilities and weaknesses are integrated into the concept of the self with greater ease and less discomfort.

Humor can also be used to develop a new viewpoint on past difficulties. The group leader, along with a supportive group, can often help a member see the humor in his or her own predicaments. Humor in an autobiography is an indication that the writer has understood, and possibly conquered, a problem. As a group evolves and its members become more experienced with the autobiographical process, humor becomes more frequent. Its use suggests that a person has moved from seeing life as a series of problems to greater insight and mastery. The important can be made funny and acceptable through the eyes of a group. Humor is a device to render the threatening, harmless. It reduces overwhelming and unspeakable anger or embarrassment to a shared laugh and to a discussable level.

Social Gains for Older Adults

In this section we discuss the importance of group experiences to the social well-being of older adults. You can play an important role in ensuring quality of life for a number of older adults by bringing them together to meet and share memories in the guided autobiography groups.

Avoiding Isolation

A key problem of the later years of life is the loss of a wife, husband, or friends and relatives. As society has moved towards nuclear families, often spread over long distances, older adults are in need of social contacts and supports outside the family. Yet, this is a period of life marked by the mortality of one's closest companions. Older people must adapt to the death of friends. The development of new late-life friendships and confidant relationships is often a by-product of participation in the guided autobiography group.

Even in families where older adults are in close proximity or living with relatives, there is a need to interact with people one's own age and to develop close friendships beyond the age-graded roles of grandparent and parent. Social isolation in the later years is associated with earlier death, increased disability, and poor mental health. Services that bring the older adult in contact with new people open the door for the development of new friendships and social support.

Guided autobiography is ideally suited to this purpose, since it builds friendships among group members. Life-long friendships are often created as the developmental exchange progresses.

In particular, for nursing home residents and others in institutional care, the move to the institution often symbolizes separation from home and society. Newly institutionalized persons may seek to further isolate themselves defensively because of depression, feelings of isolation, and fear of developing new emotional ties. The interactions afforded in the guided autobiography groups have proven to have positive outcomes for such persons, often resulting in:

- Less time spent in one's room
- The development of a few key friendships
- Increased openness to sharing one's life story
- Increased willingness to meet new people
- A change into a more interesting person for others to talk to

Confidants

Since a review of one's life is a frequent activity near the end of life, older adults are likely to engage in some form of autobiography even if no group is available. Many older adults may want to engage in life review during periods of traumatic loss (such as loss of a spouse or personal disability), but they lack a confidant.

Losses may have severe repercussions, lowering overall satisfaction and leading to depression. A negative world view, invoked by loss and depression, can elicit a preoccupation with exaggerated memories of defeat or failure over the life course. Such distortion of a life, however, may remain unidentified in the absence of persons with whom to share one's thoughts. The support and perspective provided by a guided autobiography group and other confidants can assist people in viewing their losses from the broader perspective of an entire life span, refocusing attention on gains and successes, and achieving a perspective or a balance of perceived pluses and minuses.

Cohort Interaction

Guided autobiography groups that are designed specifically for older persons can benefit individuals through their being with people one's own age. In these groups, members are able to relate easily to the past and the present of other members.

Living through similar times invokes positive shared memories of times gone by and increased understanding of how past events impacted differently on different people. Comparability of current circumstances of living can provide not only emotional support but also the opportunity for sharing adaptive strategies. For example, a group brought together as part of a program designed to facilitate adaptation to a chronic illness can provide members with an opportunity to exchange valuable information on how to manage different aspects of the illness.

Intergenerational Interaction

Often, living arrangements dictate whether homogeneous groups are formed of persons with similar experiences. These groups are particularly desirable if the goal is to facilitate adaptation to a new living environment or disability. In general, however, the authors favor heterogeneous groups when possible, since the range of experience and memories is greater and thereby enriching. Groups with members of a wide age range and many backgrounds may take longer to "gel," but they are more evocative and stronger when they coalesce.

Research indicates that beneficial effects occur when different generations relate to one another in a group setting. These include:

1. The opportunity for the young and old to act out and resolve family roles, particularly misunderstandings regarding intergenerational interactions
2. The ability to understand better the common elements and distinct perspectives of different phases we experience over our lives
3. The opportunity for older adults to act as mentors to younger persons and for younger adults to benefit from the "wisdom of years"
4. The opportunity for different generations to review and contrast their values and experiences

A mix of ages appears to add a dimension to the process that might not exist in a group whose members are similar in age. Old, young, and middle-aged adults appear to enjoy reflecting on both the similarities and differences found among the generations. The younger members of the groups often help older members understand the intergenerational relations that the older people had previously found confusing or hurtful. Older members often become surrogate parents or grandparents for the younger participants. The depth of these relationships is illustrated by the tendency of group members to keep in touch with one another long after the formal process is complete.

In a similar manner, persons of different ethnic backgrounds and careers add to the richness of the group experience. Heterogeneity in group composition should not be avoided but encouraged as much as possible by inviting men and women of diverse ages and backgrounds.

So, Why Write?

Although the group experience holds rich potential and is a valuable component of guided autobiography, writing one's autobiographical statements is also an important part of this process. The sensitization process that begins in the group is only the first step in a person's journey into a review of the self and the personal past. Personal, private reflection and the motivation to delve deeply into the banks of the memory are summoned by the task of writing down one's recollections.

In addition, the writing process itself is a stimulus to further recall. As thoughts are put on paper, rearranged, and read, related memories are elicited. The perspective of the self as a reader also provides the person with a unique opportunity to obtain a degree of separation from the material. This helps open the door for the emergence of new perspectives on the past, the perspective of the more distant and mature present.

By writing one's thoughts down before sharing them with the group, a person is, in a sense, rehearsing. He or she can plan what will be shared with the group, homing in on the experiences that were most important. Without this opportunity, the account of memories might ramble, and the person's time to share with the group might be taken up by less meaningful recall. Similarly, a person has the opportunity to review his or her life theme and determine what will and will not be shared with the group. This protects the individual's right to monitor the developmental exchange and not to share what he or she feels is too personal or painful.

Finally, without the written document, a person would have difficulty reconstructing his statements about life themes in order to later expand the autobiography if he wished to do a more comprehensive version. This would eliminate the potential of sharing his autobiographical life stories with persons outside the group and would reduce the usefulness of guided autobiography to help create a family legacy to pass on to others.

Among the most valuable gifts you can give your children and grandchildren is your life story. It can provide them with a sense of continuity and solidity that enhances the development of self-understanding. In today's era of families scattered over large regions, and even different continents, it is a way to provide one's children, grandchildren, and even great-grandchildren with a feeling that they know who you are and therefore know better who they are.

Chapter **4**

The Importance of Guiding Themes

G UIDED AUTOBIOGRAPHY is based on the conviction that certain themes form common threads that run through lives and bind the fabric of human life. The specific themes employed in guided autobiography are the result of years of development and refinement. The initial set of themes and sensitizing questions used in guided autobiography were assembled through a graduate seminar of a select group of psychologists and social scientists with backgrounds and interest in the autobiographical process. These themes and questions have been revised in response to the feedback of participants and group leaders.

What has been extracted from this process is a series of themes that have proven to be important in the lives of most people. These themes are described fully in Chapter 5 and include the major branching points in life; the family; one's career, life work, or both; the role of money in one's life; health and body image; loves and hates; sexual identity; experiences with death and other losses; aspirations and goals; and the influences, beliefs, and values that provide meaning in life.

These themes have been chosen for four fundamental reasons. First, they are powerful issues that run through the life course. Second, they demonstrate that review of one's life in this framework is beneficial in guiding next steps and in transcending crises. Third, they show that the thematic approach enhances the group process by providing a basis for sharing common feelings and circumstances. Finally, they form a meaningful legacy, since these themes are the outcomes of life experiences and issues that are relevant to other generations.

The order in which the themes are presented is designed to correspond with the successful progression of the developmental exchange. As can well be imagined, group members' willingness to share memories and feelings concerning highly personal and potent life issues, such as body image and sexual history, is conditional on the early development of trust within the group. This trust can only be acquired through the process of sharing increasingly personal information. A metaphor for this process is that of a child who tentatively wades in shallow water until acquiring the confidence and trust necessary to dive into deeper territory.

Emotional Saliency and Life Themes

Salience is defined as "a striking point or feature" denoting that which projects "above or beyond a general level" (*Webster's Third New International Dictionary*, 1981). Life issues that are emotionally salient are those that have had the strongest impact on one's emotions and that are powerful in determining a person's course of action or in shaping the identity.

The topics chosen for personal exploration and group interaction in guided autobiography are designed to focus attention and stimulate recall of memories of the formative experiences of life that are most emotionally salient. By directing attention to the emotional issues and events of life, the group leader guides participants in the search for self-understanding. The leader provides a context in which exploration and, in a sense, the retelling and reliving of important experiences open the door to greater understanding and possibly even acceptance of one's past and current feelings.

> Sam was referred to the group by a nurses' aide who hoped it would help him regain his self-esteem, which seemed to be diminishing as his physical capacity decreased because of severe arthritis. With the support of the other group members who challenged Sam to explore the techniques he was using to compensate for this disability, Sam began to see his experiences with arthritis more as a sign of his own technical ingenuity and capacity to adapt than as a sign of decreased vigor. For example, he recounted the many uses he now had for pliers, which he used to compensate for his lack of grip strength.
>
> Other group members commented about arthritis sufferers they knew who simply restricted their activities rather than applying new strategies and tools. This focused Sam's attention on his skill in this area and served as an impetus for Sam to continue finding creative ways to manage tasks.

In writing his essay on the theme of health and body image, Sam began to recognize the emotional stake he had put in his physical prowess throughout his life. This helped him understand better his own feelings about his disability.

The Role of Life Themes in Successful Transitions

The themes chosen for guided autobiography are designed to focus thoughts on the major changes and adaptations that have been made throughout the life course. Particularly in older adults, reviewing the many ways in which they have adjusted to or overcome the demands and hardships of life often provides them with a strong sense of self-esteem and competency.

The first life-story theme assigned in guided autobiography, "History of the Major Branching Points in Your Life," introduces the participants to the flow metaphor and the many factors that can influence the flow of life. In sharing descriptions of the decision processes and chance events, the individual's role is highlighted in directing the course of life. In the process, the personal strengths and skills that might otherwise be overlooked are brought to the surface. These are the key-pins for future successful transitions and adaptations.

Themes for discussion are not only the fertile choices but also those that lead to a dead-end. The ability to recognize that pursuit of a branch is fruitless, to change direction or even sever that branch, and to begin again from an earlier point is an important aspect of personal strength and adaptation. We sometimes must summon all our strength to cut off and tar over a branch that has become diseased and could damage those parts of the tree of life that have yet to bear fruit. Our ability to do this and to transcend the scars that remain is a vital aspect of our strength to survive and succeed. The following example shows the potential benefits of this process as reflected in the experience of one member of a past guided autobiography group:

> Doris, now age 70, still felt the repercussions of an early divorce on her self-esteem. At the age of 30 her marriage ended due to her ex-husband's chronic drug addiction. This addiction was the result of morphine provided in an army hospital during World War II. Doris felt that she could not blame her husband since he had suffered greatly, but she was concerned that his addiction and the associated turmoil would damage her children irrevoca-

bly. She ended the marriage in the interest of her childrens' well-being, but she saw this as a personal failure, and she blamed herself for being unable to help her husband and make the marriage work.

In addressing the theme assignment "History of Your Family," Doris wrote a great deal about her postdivorce history as a single mother, its challenges, and the ultimate successes of her two sons. Never before having put this story together in one place (or reflection), she found herself impressed by all she had accomplished as a single mother and how productive the choices she made for her sons' lives had been.

Although she still regretted her earlier inability to change her husband's circumstance, after reviewing her entire family history, Doris began to recognize more of her successes as an adaptive and caring person and to develop a more integrated, complete picture of herself to the benefit of her self-esteem.

In the context of exploring and sharing life stories based on subsequent themes, a complete picture of the "branching tree of life" unfolds. This picture, with its branches, knots, and scars, helps prepare the older adult for branches yet to be made by providing an increased sense of competence and a future orientation. (For more on these outcomes, see Chapter 1.)

Common Meeting Grounds

As was discussed in Chapter 3, an important aspect of guided autobiography is that it occurs in a group. Successful group experiences spawn many benefits:

- Support
- Acceptance
- New insights
- Availability of interested listeners
- A sense of cohesiveness and belonging
- Confidant relationships
- Camaraderie
- Empathy
- A feeling of relatedness, that you are understood partly because others are similar

A vital component of this is the enhanced ability of group members to recognize themselves in the life stories of others. The use of themes and sensitizing questions is a practical way to keep group members focusing on the same issues, increasing the opportunity for discovering similarities and differences.

The Family Legacy

Since the themes chosen elicit key life issues, they are particularly suited to lead to a written family legacy. Making available to younger generations one's thoughts and experiences, a person can present his or her family with an opportunity for intergenerational comparisons and contrasts. Also, he or she can greatly enhance the transmission of values, adaptive strategies, and details of family history.

The Use of Sensitizing Questions

In the last section we discussed the reasons for employing a thematic approach in guided autobiography. Here, we will clarify the benefits of sensitizing questions, including their role in stimulating interaction in the group and in facilitating recall and personal reflection. As described in Chapter 2, the sensitizing questions on each theme are distributed and briefly discussed at the meeting preceding the session at which the life-story essay on that theme will be read. This accomplishes two primary objectives:

1. Group members are guided through the autobiography process in a manner that builds momentum and understanding. That is, the order in which themes are addressed is controlled such that (a) the most basic issues of life (e.g., family) are dealt with first and can help inform reflection on later themes, and (b) the more sensitive issues are, for the most part, later in the process and shared with the group after trust has been built.
2. Other group members' interpretations of questions and perceptions regarding the facets of life that comprise a theme stimulate expansion of one's own perspective and promote flexibility of recall.

The primary role of sensitizing questions is to define and clarify the kinds of life events and issues that are important to a life theme. For example, take the theme "History of Your Family." Simply asked to write on this topic, a person might develop a chronology or family tree and focus on the history of distant ancestors. Another person might describe the origin of his or her family, explaining where and when they moved from place to place, describing the birth order of siblings, or providing an overview of the major accomplishments and employment histories of different family members.

These details are useful to recall, but what might be missed is reflection on the aspects of the family that shaped the individual. The sensitizing questions for this topic are designed to focus attention on the role of the family in determining the particular self. As such, they promote recall and reflection, which is emotionally salient and meaningful for increased self-understanding.

An autobiography is a personal account of a life. Sensitizing questions *guide* group members to explore aspects of their life histories that are most emotionally powerful and most closely linked to individual development—which molded the self or the identity.

Advise group members that the sensitizing questions are meant to guide but *not limit or direct* their thinking. Questions should not be addressed as a test or homework assignment to be answered. Group members should be told that some of the questions may not apply to them and that they should feel free to skip some and add others when they follow their own exploration of the topic. Finally, it should be stressed that the life-story essays should not be a series of implicit or explicit questions and answers per se. If a group member feels that he or she would gain more by taking an approach not reflected in the sensitizing questions, he or she should be encouraged to do so. With the exception of assigning themes and the two-page limit, no restrictions should be placed on personal reflection and the writing of life-story essays. The purpose of sensitization is to stimulate recall and reflection, expand perspectives, and initiate sharing.

Sensitization and Memory

The most practical reason for employing sensitizing questions is that they strengthen recall. As the group leader and other group members reflect on the sensitizing questions, which should be distributed early in each session, the vignettes of experience they relate help stimulate others to recall their experiences. The questions bring to mind stories, personalities, emotions, and events from the past that might otherwise be forgotten.

Since our purpose here is not to instruct the reader on the processes of memory, it suffices to say that memory depends upon stimuli, a present event, thought, or mood that provokes recall of related past memories. Returning to the metaphor of the fisherman, just as the use of themes serves as a map to the best fishing holes, the use of sensitizing questions serves as appropriate bait to attract the biggest fish (most relevant memories).

Evolving Perspectives

Guided autobiography is based on the belief that exploring one's life story has direct and indirect healing powers. The process can greatly enhance the present well-being of older adults who actively engage in the process. Further, it is based on the conviction that the *productive* recall of past experiences is a result of *systematic reminiscence,* defined as purposeful, directed attention to how one's life and the self have been shaped. This is in contrast to spontaneous reminiscence, which is the recall of aspects of our past with limited or no purpose or organization; this type of recall is exemplified by our random daily conversations.

The use of sensitizing questions increases awareness of the many ways a given life theme can be approached. The awareness is further enhanced by discussion of the themes and their sensitizing questions in the group before personal reflection and writing. Discussion promotes an evolution of thought as members examine their histories from a variety of vantage points, searching for an angle that sheds the most light.

Thus, we employ sensitizing questions as a means to expand perspectives and productively channel attention to each theme in guided autobiography.

Group Discussion and Sensitization

Along with an expanded perspective stimulated by group interaction about a given theme, there is the further benefit of promoting the developmental exchange through the use of sensitizing questions. Developmental exchange is the escalating process of trading personal stories with another person.

As was described, the use of themes and sensitizing questions provides a "common meeting ground" that fosters feelings of cohesiveness, empathy, and relatedness; in short, their use gives members the belief that they are understood and accepted. This helps build the trust that is so vital to the progression of the developmental exchange and its benefits (see Chapter 3).

The use of sensitizing questions also serves as a guide for the group leader in estimating where members are in the continuum of the developmental exchange. The progression of themes poses more and more emotionally salient questions. In this manner, there is an ongoing expansion of the personal information that is shared in the group. This is not meant either to limit interaction or to compel members to share more than is comfortable.

Exploration of the sensitizing questions has been found to provide a comfortable framework that encourages members to proceed into deeper and deeper territory by allowing them to do so in stages. This approach is sensitive to the needs people have to test the waters and develop security at one level before progressing to the next. By sharing some of their thoughts during the preliminary discussion, members also get a sense of each other's investment in the developmental exchange. This helps members gauge their own comfort levels as they progressively share openly and productively, while at the same time withholding information that they do not want to share.

Chapter 5

Successful Themes and Sensitizing Questions

PARTICULARLY for older adults and others in transition, writing and sharing one's autobiography is a big step forward in integrating and developing a sense of direction in one's life. At any age and at any transition phase in life, doing one's autobiography can yield meaning and a sense of acceptance and of peace. Autobiography is not an end in itself but a beginning of the future, a future that will unfold better if we have a clearer view of the past. As noted in Chapter 4, certain themes elicit the most salient memories and therefore are best suited for the autobiographical process. In addition, questions can be asked in the context of such themes to sensitize the participants to the possible issues, further enhancing the elicitation of memories.

The following materials are the specific themes and sensitizing questions that generally have been used in conducting guided autobiography groups. Additional themes and questions might be added, particularly in groups that are formed based on a common context or concern, for example, retired physicians, recent nursing home residents, recovering addicts. As noted earlier, the sensitizing questions are not meant to restrict the process. Preliminary discussion of a given theme may be beneficial, given its potential to expand sensitization and open the participant to possible new perspectives.

Theme Assignment 1: The Major Branching Points in Your Life

Think of your life as a branching tree, as a flowing river that has many juncture points, or as a trailing plant that puts down roots at various places and then grows on.

What is a branching point? Branching points are events, experiences, or happenings in our lives that significantly affect the direction or flow of our life. Branching points are experiences that shape our lives in some important way.

Branching points may be big events (e.g., marriage, retirement, geographical move) or they may seem small and apparently inconsequential (e.g., reading a book, going on a hike). Big outcomes may have small beginnings.

From your point of view, what were the major branching points in your life? What were the events, experiences, interactions with people and places that had a major influence or impact on the way your life has flowed?

Sensitizing Questions

1. About how old were you at the time of the branching point? Place the turning point along a time dimension. The timing of an event is often very important. Did it happen too soon? Were you too young? Did it happen too late? Were you too old?

2. Significant people? Who were the important people involved in the turning point? Father, mother, spouse? You alone? Often one notices that the same people are involved again and again in major life turning points.

3. Emotions and feelings at that time? What were the feelings, the emotions you experienced at the time the branching point occurred? How intense were these feelings (e.g., extremely elated, somewhat sad, a little frustrated, very happy)? Sometimes our feelings in reaction to an experience are mixed or are changeable. Do not be concerned if your feelings seem contradictory.

4. Emotions and feelings now? Sometimes our feelings about an experience or event change over time. Something that seemed a disaster when it happened may turn out to be a positive event later on and vice versa. What emotions do you experience as you think about the turning point now?

5. Personal choice? How much personal choice was involved in this branching point? How much personal control did you have? Was it something that happened that was completely out of your control? Who or what was the external influence?

6. Consequences? Branching points are "branching points" because they change our lives in one or many important ways. In your

view, what are the ways your life was changed because of this branching point? What effect, impact, consequences did it have on your life? How would your life have been different if it had not occurred?

Theme Assignment 2: Your Family

What is your family? The history of your family includes your family of origin (among them, grandparents, parents, siblings, uncles and aunts) as well as your family of adulthood (among them, spouse, children, grandchildren).

The family members important in shaping your life should be mentioned, not necessarily all the family members. Some have been more important in positive ways and some in negative ways in shaping your life.

What family members have had a major impact in shaping your life? Why?

What would another person have to know about your family in order to understand you and how you've come to be the person you are?

Sensitizing Questions

1. Who held the power in your family? Why? Who made the decisions? How did you know?
2. Who offered support, warmth, and nurturance? Why? Who did you go to for comfort? Who did you confide in?
3. What major family member(s) have you been closest to? Why?
4. What important family member did you know the least? Feel least close to? Why? Who should you have been close to but for some reason were not?
5. Did you like your family? Why or why not?
6. What was best about your family? Worst about it? What were (are) the strengths and weaknesses in your family?
7. Was there anyone in your family you were afraid of? Why?
8. Who were the heroes in your family? The family favorites? How did you know?
9. What was the feeling tone in your family (e.g., happy, sad, crowded, spacious, noisy, quiet, warm, cold)?
10. What were the major areas of conflict, problems, and issues in your family?
11. What were the rules in your family, the "shoulds" and "oughts"?

12. What events and experiences have torn your family apart or have made your family stronger?
13. Were you loved? How did you know?

Theme Assignment 3: Your Major Life Work or Career

What is a career? It is your major life's work. It occupies your energy, your activity, and your time. A career, a life work, can have many forms. Usually we think of it as work outside the home for pay. A life work can also be found in being a husband, a wife, a parent, or in religious devotion, in play, in art, in education, in community service. This does not necessarily involve a salary or pay. People can have a number of careers, a sequence of careers, or both.

What has been your major life's work or career?

Sensitizing Questions

1. How did you get into your major life work? How did you find it? Did you choose it because your family expected it? Was it because of a teacher you knew? Did your appearance have anything to do with it? When did you begin your life work?
2. How early did you formulate your life career goals? What did you want to be when you grew up? How have childhood interests, passions, teachers influenced the path your life work has taken? How much choice did you have?
3. What has been the developmental course of your life work? Has it been continuous? Discontinuous? What have been the peaks and valleys? Have there been major or minor setbacks? Major changes in focus? Have you had a sequence or series of careers?
4. What have been the biggest influences in directing the path of your career once chosen? For example, have they been people, places, events?
5. If you do not have a major life work (yet), what would you like to do? Why?
6. If you feel you have finished your major life work, how do you evaluate it?
7. How has your work provided new options? Limited options?
8. Are you "on time" in your career, or ahead or behind in terms of your expectations?

9. What have been (are) the challenges of your life work? Your successes? The problems? The failures?
10. If you have more than one life-work identity, which of these has been the most important to you? Why?
11. What has been unique or special about your work experiences? Place of work? Travel? People?
12. What have you enjoyed most about your life work? Least?
13. If you had it to do over again, how would you develop differently along your life-work path? Would you choose the same life work? Why or why not?

Theme Assignment 4: The Role of Money in Your Life

Money is one of the most important themes in life. It is both an obvious and a subtle influence. Money touches many aspects of our lives—family, education, career, health, relationships with others, and self-esteem.

Your attitude towards money has been shaped by many influences, both positive and negative.

Sensitizing Questions

1. What role did money play in your family? What were you taught about money? Was it scarce or plentiful? Were you poor or well off?
2. How did your family's money compare to other people's money?
3. In your life, how important is it to make money?
4. Does money have any relationship to love in your life? How?
5. What was the first time you earned any money? How did you feel about it? How did it affect your later ideas about money?
6. What have been your greatest financial successes?
7. What have been your worst financial mistakes?
8. How central is the role that money plays in your life?
9. Does money have any relationship to your self-esteem?
10. How much do you think about money? Do you worry about money?
11. Do you regard yourself as generous or stingy? Why?
12. Have you ever borrowed money? How did you feel about it?
13. Are you a good or a poor manager of money? Why?
14. Do you ever give money away? How do you feel about it?

Theme Assignment 5: Your Health and Body Image

The image of your body and your health has many aspects, objective features, and subjective feelings. In part, it involves an implied comparison with other persons, whether you were (are) more or less healthy, stronger or weaker, coordinated or clumsy, attractive or unattractive. How do you regard your body and health?

What has been the history of your health and body image?

Sensitizing Questions

1. What was your health like as a baby? As a child? Adolescent? Young adult? Middle-aged adult? Older adult?
2. Were you considered a sickly child? If so, what were the consequences for your development?
3. Were you a fast-developing or slow-developing child? Were you ahead or behind in growth as an adolescent?
4. What health problems have you experienced in your life? How did you feel about each of these? How did you handle these problems?
5. How has your body reacted to games and athletic sports?
6. In what ways does your body react to stress? Has this changed during your life? What do you do in response to your body's stress signals?
7. What have you done during your life to help/hurt your health?
8. How would you describe your physical appearance as a baby? Child? Adolescent? Young adult? Middle-aged adult? Older adult? Are (were) you short, tall, thin, fat, attractive, ugly, poised, awkward?
9. What part(s) of your body do you like least? Why? How has this changed over your life?
10. What part(s) of your body do you like most? Why? How has this changed over your life?
11. What have you done to alter, change, or improve your health and physical self during your life?
12. How do you regard your body in terms of female or male image?
13. If you could change your body in any way, how would you want it to be different?

Theme Assignment 6: Your Sexual Identity, Sex Roles, and Sexual Experiences

Sexuality includes our sense of ourselves as male or female (sexual identity), our ideas about appropriate sex role behavior, and our sexual experiences.

What has been the history of your sexual development, including the development of your identity as male/female, your concepts of appropriate sex role behavior, your sexual experiences?

Sensitizing Questions

1. When did you first learn/realize that your were a boy or a girl? When did you first realize that little boys and girls were different? How did you feel about that?
2. What toys did you use and what games did you play when you were a child? Were any kinds of play, toys, games forbidden? What clothes were you dressed in as a child? What significance did this have in the development of your sexual identity?
3. Were you a "tomboy"? A "sissy"? A "fraidy cat"? Did you ever wish you had been born the opposite sex? Why?
4. What did your parents, teachers, relatives teach you about what "good" girls and boys did and did not do? What were the rules for being a boy or a girl? What were your parents' views about your sexuality?
5. Where did you get your sex education (from parents, friends, books, school, religious training)? Where and when did you learn the facts of life?
6. What were your early sexual experiences (such as doctor-and-nurse games)? Did you have childhood sweethearts?
7. Have you had any traumatic sexual experiences?
8. What have been your concepts or models of the "ideal" man or the "ideal" woman? How have these ideas changed as you have grown up and grown older?
9. What are your concepts about the "ideal" relationship between two people?
10. How would you characterize yourself as a man or woman? How has this changed? What "traditionally" masculine or feminine aspects can you identify in yourself?

11. How do you relate to members of the opposite sex? How has this changed?
12. What has been the history of your sexual experiences? How have they changed as you've grown older? What factors (e.g., aging, health, menopause, or retirement) have affected your sexual identity and sexual experiences?
13. How do you feel about your sexuality? Have your ideas about appropriate sexual behavior changed over time (e.g., attitudes toward homosexuality)?

Theme Assignment 7: Your Experiences with Death or Your Ideas about Death

Death can affect your life in many ways. You may have experienced the loss of a beloved pet as a child; you may have lost parents, grandparents, dear friends, a spouse, a child, a brother or sister. Maybe the death of a political hero affected you profoundly.

How have your experiences with death affected your life and your character? How have your reactions to death changed over the years? How have your ideas concerning your own death changed?

Sensitizing Questions

1. How did you feel about death when you were a child? Did you lose an animal that was like a member of the family? What did you think when your pet died?
2. How was death talked about and treated in your family? Did it frighten you? How did you understand it?
3. When did you go to your first funeral? How did you react?
4. What effect did the threat of death in wartime have on you?
5. Were you ever so sick you thought you might die?
6. What have been the close calls with death? Have your ideas about your own death changed over the years? How do you feel about your death now?
7. How have you grieved?
8. Do dead parents, grandparents, spouses, or others continue to have an effect on your life?
9. Do you feel guilty about anyone's death? Helpless? Angry? Resentful? Abandoned? Have you ever felt responsible for anyone's death?

10. Have you ever killed anyone? How did you feel about it at the time? How do you feel about it now?
11. Did some great person's death (e.g., Kennedy or Roosevelt) have an effect on you?
12. Is death an enemy or friend for you? Is it to be dreaded and fought, or welcomed?
13. What kind of death would you like to have?
14. If you could talk to a dead person, what would you ask him or her?
15. What was the most significant death you have experienced? How did it change you or your life?

Theme Assignment 8: Your Loves and Hates

Love is a strong emotional attachment to a particular person, place, or thing. Absence of the love object causes distress in the form of loneliness, anxiety, and longing. What have been the major loves of your life?

Hate is a strong feeling of dislike or ill will toward some person, place, or thing. What have been the hates or strong aversions in your life?

Sensitizing Questions

1. What persons, places, or things aroused your greatest feelings of love when you were a child?
2. Who was your first love?
3. Who in your life made you feel loved and why?
4. Were you ever consumed by love? When and under what circumstances?
5. What has been the role of love in your life? How has it changed over time?
6. Why did your loves end? What happens when you lose a love? Did your feelings change or did you lose the object of your love?
7. How have your ideas about love changed during your life?
8. What have been the major hates of your life? What places, people, events, characteristics of people, objects, ideas, or kinds of behavior cause you to feel extreme dislike?
9. What were your major dislikes as a child? How did they change with time?
10. Have you ever hated someone so much you wished they would die?

11. How have you expressed your hatred?
12. Have your hates changed over the years, or have they remained the same?
13. If you could wish ill upon some person by voodoo or magic, who would it be?
14. Do you express your hate or keep it inside?
15. Do you have some strong unexpressed feelings of love for some person, place, or thing?
16. When you were growing up, what were you taught about love and hate? How have your ideas changed?

Theme Assignment 9: The Meaning of Your Life, and Your Aspirations and Life Goals

Questions of meaning, values, morality, and religion are often elusive and difficult to articulate. Human life is characterized by moral complexity and ambiguity. Often the black and white of childhood, the simple delineation of right and wrong, changes to large areas of grey in our adult lives. Questions of value and meaning, religion and morality, are often fraught with contradictions. Some people become moral gymnasts, stretching and bending with agility in the moral realm of life. Others find their home in a traditional religious philosophy and structure. Numerous people today claim to have "their own religion," an eclectic synthesis of many diverse elements. Still others avow atheism or agnosticism. Secular humanism claims a large following in contemporary culture.

How do your life goals fit into your beliefs and values? How have you set your life goals? What are they? Trace the history of your moral or religious development. How has it changed through your life? Do you have a philosophy of life? What is it? What does your life mean? What does human life in general mean?

Sensitizing Questions

1. What kinds of different goals do you have—material, social, personal, universal, moral, religious—and how important are they to you? Have your goals always been the same?
2. Were there any religious traditions in your home as a child? Have you carried them on? Why or why not?
3. Have you ever had a religious experience? What were you doing and where did it happen? How did you react?

4. What symbols, either religious or secular, are significant for you? Why?
5. What are the principles that guide your life? What are your standards? What does it mean if you do not live up to them?
6. What has been your purpose in life? Have you had more than one purpose? How has this purpose (or these purposes) changed?
7. Do you find meaning in the idea of social justice, posterity, or the brotherhood of man? How do you act on these ideas?
8. Do you want to emulate some great figure (e.g., Moses, Gandhi, Christ, Schweitzer, Eleanor Roosevelt)? Who are your moral heroes? Have they changed over time?
9. Were you taught not to be cruel to animals so that you would not be cruel to people? What is your relationship to the natural world?
10. Have you ever found life meaningless? Did it fill you with despair? Did you come to some understanding?
11. Why be moral? WHY BE?

Elective Theme Assignment 10: The Role of Music, Art, or Literature in Your Life

The aesthetic aspects of our lives are sometimes obvious, sometimes subtle. Music can be the background to our daily lives, or it can be a powerful expression of a personal philosophy. Literature entertains us, instructs us, inspires us. Art may be simply decoration for some people; for others, it may play a central role in life. In this assignment you are to describe the aesthetic aspects of your life—your relationships with music, art, and literature.

Sensitizing Questions

1. Do certain pieces of music evoke memories of times past? Are they connected with old relationships? Happier times? Times of struggle?
2. What does music do to you emotionally? Do you use music to alter your mood?
3. How do you feel when you listen to religious music?
4. How do you feel when you hear patriotic music?
5. Does music touch you? Is music important to you?

6. Do you play any musical instruments? Would you like to? Why?
7. What is your favorite piece of music? Why? What does it mean to you?
8. What literary works have had an effect on your life? Can you think of books that have been important in shaping your personality or your ideas about the world? What were they?
9. Do you enjoy reading? How much or how little do you read? What kind of reading do you do?
10. Can you think of one book, essay, story, poem that had a powerful effect on you?
11. Do you ever reread things? What are they? Why do you reread them?
12. Is literature important to you? Why or why not?
13. How do you feel about art? Is it important to you? What kinds of art? Do you own any art? Would you like to?
14. Do you go to museums? Do you go to art exhibits? Do you like folk art? Classical art? Modern art? Functional art? Why?
15. Are you an artist? What kind? What does it mean to you to be an artist?

Elective Theme Assignment 11: Your Experiences with Stress

What is stress? Stress is some event that requires adaptation. It may result from a natural disaster, personal crises of various kinds (e.g., health, finances, work), or chronic hassles (e.g., housework, freeways, noise).

From your point of view, what have been the major stresses in your life? How have you coped with each stress that has come along? What have been the consequences of stress for your life and development?

Sensitizing Questions

1. How have you known you were stressed? What were the clues? What body signs or symptoms do you develop when you are under stress? Have these symptoms changed as you have grown older? Are you more sensitive to these signs now?
2. What have been the continuing or chronic stresses in your life? Intermittent stresses? Short-lived stresses?
3. How have your ways of coping with stress changed? How did you cope as a child? Adolescent? Young adult? Middle-aged adult? Older adult?

4. Who were the models for coping with stress in your life (e.g., what did you learn about coping from parents, teachers, peers)? How did you learn to cope with stress? What were (are) the "rules" for coping with stress?
5. Were there important people in your life who helped you recognize and cope with stress?
6. How does your feeling of personal control affect your reaction to stress? What about self-induced stress? Stress over which you have no control?
7. Under what circumstances do you collapse and become unable to cope with stress? What kinds of stress do you find overwhelming? Has this changed as you have grown older?
8. What have been the consequences of stress in your life? Positive ones? Negative ones?

Chapter 6

Encouraging Creativity
and Divergent Thinking

M ANY PEOPLE do not view themselves as creative and may therefore be reluctant to experiment in writing their life stories. Yet, these same people can often knit beautiful garments, refinish furniture, or create a garden that far surpasses the average row of flowers. To awaken the creative potential in others may simply require drawing their attention to the many modes of creative expression and to the ways in which they have been creative in their own right. Everyday signs of creative expression may be seen in

sewing, needlework, and crocheting
woodworking
cooking
gardening
problem solving
entrepreneurial endeavors
playing an instrument
inventing, constructing, or integrating many other ideas and
materials

Creativity is behavior that results in new functions, forms, or ideas. A creative act does not imitate or repeat the old but generates novelty that can be judged to represent a desirable innovation. Creativity involves flexibility of mind, fluency or the flow of ideas, and originality. Breaking of old concepts or looking at things in a new way is a component of creativity called *divergent thinking*. One can show divergent thinking in looking at old problems in new ways.

Creativity in adults is believed to be the counterpart of play in children (Kaminsky, 1978). Kaminsky suggested that remembering the past itself might be described as "a valuable and creative form of play, an activity which is its own reward" (p. 21). Playfulness in approach to events in our past during the guided autobiography process can open the door to new perspectives and insights into one's life stories. Playfulness is a necessary component of humor and is yet another link that binds group members. Humor shows divergent thinking, or creativity, since it involves looking at old, often stereotyped situations in new ways, for example, the statement "autobiography is a story of a man's life told by his worst enemy."

Creative expression expands a person's view of the world and provides alternatives. It can also be a highly enjoyable aspect of participating in guided autobiography. Not unlike humor, creative metaphors and poetry are ways of expressing indirectly that which might be difficult to express directly in more conventional ways. Through the creative exercise, a person can gain distance from the emotionally difficult and develop an increased sense of mastery.

Divergent thinking moves in different directions from a familiar or conventional point of view. This is in contrast to *convergent thinking*, which represents movement to a single conclusion, with the assumption that there is one and only one correct answer to a question. For example, if asked to describe the use of a paper clip, the convergent thinker would say that it is used to hold papers together. The divergent thinker would include this among a (potentially limitless) number of alternative uses, which might include such responses as:

"I could bend it into a hook for fishing."
"It could be straightened and used to jimmy a lock."
"I could bend it into an animal to make a toy."
"It could be linked to other paper clips to make a bracelet or
    necklace."
"I could use it to hold together two pieces of cloth."

Here, the thinker is exploring novel avenues and allowing his or her thoughts to flow from one possible use of the paper clip to another. The process is creative, generating new and more powerful solutions to problems or supplying new perspectives on the familiar.

Creativity and the Older Adult

The healthy human brain continues to store information over the entire life span (Birren, 1990). Thus, one's vocabulary is greater at age 65 than it is at age 25, as much as twice as large. Well-functioning older adults store more experience or information in their nervous systems than their young counterparts. Their histories also afford them alternative strategies and styles of problem solving that they have employed and observed over time. All things being equal, it then should follow that older adults can use this greater information and experiential base as a springboard for the creative process.

All things, however, are not equal over the life span. With age can come stereotyped or rigid ways of viewing oneself and others. Also, increases in stored information are counterbalanced by slowing of information processing (Ruth and Birren, 1985); an increased cautiousness in older persons' willingness to risk new solutions (Botwinick, 1978); and social influences such as role- and job-related pressures, which discourage older adults from thinking divergently and behaving creatively (Berg and Ruth, 1982). Indeed, possibly as a result of such influences, researchers have found that creativity declines with age (Alpaugh and Birren, 1977). As yet, it is not clear whether creativity inevitably declines with age or whether the trend toward convergent thinking is a consequence of long-term adaptations to a career, relations to family, and community roles such that the capacity to be creative is unused and shows disuse atrophy.

A person who has a highly creative orientation throughout the life course, despite age-related declines, may well remain more creative in his or her later years than many younger people who show little creativity.

Furthermore, social influences, as reflected in society's too frequent dismissal of older adults as "set in their ways" and obsolete, can themselves be neutralized by social support and interest. Excessive cautiousness might dissipate or even turn to playfulness in an atmosphere of acceptance and encouragement.

By promoting creativity and divergent thinking during the guided autobiography process, you as the group leader encourage the participant to expand his or her perspective. The use of creative devices can also awaken memories and emotions that might otherwise be forgotten. For some participants, the first step in this process is conquering the fear of writing.

Conquering the Fear of Writing

Many older adults and others feel reluctant to participate in a program that requires them to write. For some, this concern is based on a feeling that they have received insufficient formal education. Others are self-conscious about their ability to write well or to have something interesting to say. The first step in conquering this reluctance is to assure potential participants that (1) the guided autobiography process is not a course on writing; (2) no one in the group need actually read all of what he or she has written, since only the two-page life stories are shared orally with the group; (3) there will be no criticism of style or correction of grammar, and spelling does not matter; and (4) nothing is more interesting to others than the details of people's lives.

For those who are uneasy without instructions or who request a few guidelines about how to write their life stories, we suggest the following:

1. In writing your autobiography, write in a "story style," write as you speak. Do not attempt to write a polished essay or piece of literature. The purpose of guided autobiography is to organize your life story and share it with others. The intent is to develop a better understanding of yourself; therefore the written word should sound like *you*. For those who plan to use their life stories to create and pass on a family legacy, children and grand-children will benefit more from a legacy that properly reflects the person and people behind it than from a well-written, nonpersonal historical account. It is the person's own voice that moves people and provides the most meaningful insights.

2. Put in details, such as descriptions of colors and odors you might recall or favorite family phrases. "Do you remember the smell of baking bread?" These highly personal memories provide the texture for the fabric of life and make it "real" for other group members and your family.

3. Write things down as you recall them; they can be reorganized later if you desire a running chronological account, a more thematic presentation, or a story told as flashbacks.

4. Include your feelings; the facts may be less important than how you felt and feel about them.

5. Generalizations about your life are important, but the recounting of vivid incidents anchors these generalizations and promotes understanding.

6. Write openly. Feel free to reveal successes and transgressions, strengths and weaknesses, and feelings of affection and ill will. Remember, not all the written information needs to be shared with the group or retained in a version designed as a family legacy.

7. To sharpen your memory, you might look at old photographs, letters, or souvenirs. Some participants find that half the fun of

guided autobiography is its power to motivate them to contact old friends and distant family to "relive" times past.

8. If you can not remember a name or date, do not let it distract you. Describe what you can and go on with the writing. You may get the missing date or name later.

9. Allow the themes and sensitizing questions to guide but not structure your thinking. Do not attempt to answer all the sensitizing questions, and realize that some may not apply to you. They were designed to stimulate memory and your thinking about your life.

10. Humorous incidents can often be as important to understanding the self as the traumatic events of the life. In retrospect, many hardships can appear humorous. Funny stories about oneself or relatives and ancestors can help to illustrate the context of personal development.

Some group members may require assistance in the writing process; for example, blind participants or the illiterate may be unable to write their thematic life stories. The group leader can recommend the recruitment of a family member, care provider, or friend to write down the person's recollections. Alternatively, since the reason for writing is to provide an opportunity for private reflection and, if desired, to create a legacy, there is the option of taping a person's life stories. The audiotape will serve all the purposes of the written word, with one exception: when sharing the story with the group, the member will need to rely on his or her memory of what was said rather than on a written document. Replay of tapes in a group is not recommended, since it detracts from the interaction of the speaker and the group.

The Use of Self-descriptive Words

As noted in Chapter 1, self-descriptive words tell us how a person defines his or her identity. Guided autobiography has been found to result in changes in the self-descriptive words chosen by the participants. This can occur as a natural by-product of the changed view of the self and the increased self-understanding that results from the process.

Promoting the expansion or reorientation of the self-concept as reflected in the use of self-descriptive words is an expression of creativity and divergent thinking released by the process. One way to demonstrate this is to ask the members at the first session to write down ten words that best describe themselves. Then ask them to number in order the three most descriptive words. After finishing their lists, they are asked to share some of these with the group. The group leader writes the different members' self-descriptive words on a blackboard if available. In past guided autobiography groups, self-descriptive words shared in this manner have ranged from terms that describe roles, such as "mother," to personal qualities, such as "ambitious."

The different nature of such descriptive words and their implications are then explored. The leader should give emphasis to the kind of words used (e.g., nouns, verbs) and the different orientations they reflect (e.g., positive or negative traits). Through exploration of self-descriptive words, group members can learn new ways of thinking about the self. A second list of ten words can be generated by each member at a later session, preferably the last session of the guided autobiography meetings.

The two lists of self-descriptive words that follow are provided for comparison and contrast. Both lists were generated by a 62-year-old woman who participated in the guided autobiography process. The first was written at the initial meeting of the group, the second, after four meetings.

First List	*Second List*
Mother	Mother
Wife	Woman
Woman	Caring
Old	Intelligent
Tall	Zestful
Overweight	Innovative
Intelligent	Kind
Thoughtful	Success
Caring	Daughter
Nurturing	Hot pink

Here, we see a shift from an emphasis on roles and the physical self to an emphasis on the personal qualities of the self. The inclusion of the word "daughter" is most likely a result of the recent experience of exploring family history, which may have reawakened the individual to the important role being a daughter, and a particular person's daughter, played in her life. The inclusion of the descriptive word "hot pink" demonstrates the ways in which divergent thinking is encouraged, in that it conveys a new approach to self-evaluation, that is more metaphorical in thinking.

The Use of Metaphors

Related to self-descriptive words are the metaphors we use to describe ourselves or our lives. A metaphor is a "figure of speech in which a word or phrase denoting one kind of object or action is used in place of another to suggest a likeness or analogy between them"; here, an analogy refers to a "resemblance in some particulars between things otherwise unalike" (*Webster's Third New International Dictionary*, 1981).

An apt metaphor is useful in understanding one's life; it can express meanings in a short phrase or even a word that might otherwise take a book to explain. "I have been a pussycat all my life, but now I am becoming a tigress," one woman said with a smile, and the guided autobiography group smiled with her. This demonstrates how the complex can be grasped through the apt metaphor.

There are three elements in a metaphor: (1) cognition, that is, the metaphor refers to something; (2) affect, it reflects our feelings about the "thing"; and (3) connation, it reflects our motivation. A person calling him- or herself a "workhorse" is clearly balancing these three elements in picking that particular descriptive word. Terms like mule, deer, or bull all suggest different relations between the three basic elements of a metaphor.

Creativity is involved in producing new metaphors for familiar as well as vaguely known persons and things. Science is thought to use root metaphors in its explanations. Shifts in scientific thought reflect new root metaphors that have elements of information, affect, and motivation embedded in them. How do we judge a better from a poorer metaphor? The better metaphor is more integrative; it refers to a broader range of explanation or description; it is more general or more powerful. Another way of looking at a good metaphor is to judge how well it fits. Does it somehow seem apt? If a member of an autobiography group tells another he seems to be like an eagle, he might laugh and say, "But I always thought of myself as a crow, picking up what was left over. I never soared."

In this previous example, the descriptive metaphor of the eagle carries with it implications of power, freedom; the eagle is an animal to be reckoned with. There is much to be learned from the root metaphors we use in describing ourselves and the changes in them as we broaden the scope of life we refer to and the feeling tones expressed. For this reason, the group leader is encouraged to explore with the group the metaphors used in autobiographical writing.

"Trade in and trade up the old metaphors that you use to characterize yourselves," we tell our guided autobiography groups. One of the outcomes of guided autobiography is greater understanding and increased self-esteem. Participants see more positive relationships between themselves and their personal worlds.

Like humor, metaphors can be used to express mastery, understanding, and even reconciliation of how one has fallen short of the ideal self.

> This brings to mind a man of 65 years who, after writing on the theme of "health and body image," told the guided autobiography group that he had always wanted to be a Porsche, "slick, fast, eminently attractive, and powerful." Instead, he explained, he had ended up as he began, a Ford. The group leader asked how this made him feel, and he replied: "I always dreamed of myself as the Porsche and measured how far I was from it. Now I understand myself as the Ford and can see its good qualities: I may not be slick, but I have always functioned dependably, needed few repairs, and I get where I need to go."

The inclusion of the reliable-Ford metaphor in an autobiography not only can help to characterize a life but also seems to summarize it in a very human way. As a group leader, you can promote the exploration of metaphors and encourage your group members to trade up their old metaphors for ones that might better express the sense of their lives as a whole and more positively express their strengths. One exercise is to ask the group members to describe themselves as animals and to use this metaphor to explore the differences between the real, ideal, and public selves. The following are the steps in this exercise:

1. Ask the group: "What animal do you most resemble, not only in physical appearance, but in affect, style, and status?"
2. Once each member has responded, you might then ask: "What kind of animal do you think your friends and family would say you resemble?" Again, allow the group to respond and provide an opportunity for a brief discussion of the possible reasons for differences in perception.
3. Next ask: "What animal would you most like to resemble?" After each member responds, you might explore what changes would have to be made in order to resemble the ideal "animal" and whether these changes are viewed as possible or even favorable.
4. As a follow-up, you might repeat this exercise later in the series of group meetings and explore any changes that have occurred.

It is apparent that the group alternates its focus on the ideal, actual, and public selves. This helps the group become more divergent in thinking. Different people find different metaphors more obvious and easier to apply to themselves. For example, the previous exercise might be difficult for a person who has had little experience or knowledge of animals or who does not particularly like animals. This exercise could be applied to any type of metaphor. The following is a list of some metaphors that have been used in past guided autobiography groups:

- Animals (e.g., lion, pussycat, turtle)
- Cars (e.g., sports car, station wagon, "hot rod")
- Birds (e.g., eagle, vulture, canary, dove)
- Foods (e.g., cream puff, brussels sprouts, mashed potatoes)
- Trees (e.g., redwood, oak, weeping willow)
- Flowers (e.g., sunflower, rose, dandelion)
- Buildings (e.g., house, skyscraper, barn)
- Bodies of water (e.g., lake, stream, ocean)

The Use of Poetry

I can't tell you
But I'll try:
This is the business of a poem,
Trying to tell what you can't.
(Summers, 1970)

Poetry can be used in a number of ways in the guided autobiography process. As a group leader, you can encourage participants to integrate poetry into their writing of the two-page life stories. Original poems can be written by group members to capture a phase of their lives and express ideas and feelings that might otherwise be difficult to write about directly. Favorite poems can be included that reflect a person's opinions or that serve as a summarizing or integrating metaphor for events and emotions. You can introduce poetry, which may be new to the group, as part of the sensitization process or for discussion of developmental stages or common experiences. Reading a poem about childhood can provide a flashback to long-forgotten aspirations and happenings.

Poetry Written by Group Members

Although the guided autobiography process is not intended as a course in creative writing, it is an opportunity to experiment with different forms of creative expression and expand our characterizations of ourselves. Since there are no critiques of style or assessments of talent and since trust is built through the group's acceptance and support, group members may feel free to explore their creative potentials in their autobiographical writings without self-conscious concerns.

You as the leader can encourage this expression by discussing the many forms the two-page life stories can take. Let group members know that past participants in the process have often chosen to write a poem about a meaningful experience or have included love poems written by or to them as part of their life histories.

When a group member includes a poetic style (e.g., the use of rhymes or a colorful metaphoric description) in his or her life stories, future attempts can be encouraged by remarks about the writing. Use simple statements that support the use of creative expression without commenting on the poem's literary value, such as: "Your metaphor of the bird made me understand a great deal in only a few words" or "The music in your rhyme really expressed your emotions during the experience."

If the group is not reluctant to try poetry, you might suggest that each member choose one life story and write a poem about it. Emphasize that the poem can be joyful, sad, or funny. Bring examples of poetic styles, including sonnets, haiku, and limericks. Stress that a poem need not rhyme. Finally, note that poetry should be used as an option, not an assignment. The best life story is written in a form with which the writer feels comfortable.

As Hollis Summers stated in his poem that began this section, "the business of a poem [is] trying to tell what you can't." Poetry can help people by putting some protective distance between their present selves and their life stories. Meaningful ideas and depths of emotion might be expressed that they might otherwise be unable to put into words or view as overly melodramatic or too revealing. Creative enterprises in the process of the guided autobiography exercise our minds and can awaken new interests and competencies, further encouraging the development of greater self-esteem in the older adult.

Poems and Sensitization

Group members should also be invited to share their favorite poems with the group. In his book on poetry therapy, psychiatrist Jack Leedy (1969) discusses the emotional gains that can accrue through the reading and sharing of poetry in a group experience. Poetry can have a cathartic effect. By definition, poetry is "writing that formulates a concentrated imaginative awareness of experience in language chosen and arranged to create a specific emotional response through its meaning, sound, and rhythm" (*Webster's Third New International Dictionary*, 1981). It is intended to touch its readers deeply, to strike a chord of common human emotion, and to contemplate aspects of the human condition with honesty and sincerity.

As such, poetry brings to awareness feelings and incidents from the past that might otherwise be forgotten. Tears are shed and the group is united through sharing a common emotional experience. For example, a poem about a first love can awaken in older adults memories and sentiments that may have long been forgotten—the scenes and emotions of youth can be revisited through the eyes and voice of the poet. As a group leader, you can stimulate this process by sharing with the group poems you have collected. Poems can be chosen that relate to the themes of the two-page life stories. An appropriate poem can be read and discussed to initiate the process of sensitization for a given theme.

Experimenting with Other Senses

Memories can be aroused by nonverbal cues as well as by the written or spoken word. How many of us are vividly reminded of a favorite grandmother by the smell of her dusting powder or perfume, or reminded of the out-of-door freedom in childhood by the odor of fresh-cut grass? Likewise, the aroma of fresh-baked bread, a Thanksgiving turkey, or baklava might bring us back to holidays long ago or to dinners with family members long departed.

The sound of an old tune can bring to mind images of ourselves at a high-school dance or remind us of the hardships of the Depression or periods of war. As a group leader you can stimulate the senses to heighten the recall and the enjoyment derived from the guided autobiography process. We will now discuss some of the materials that can be incorporated into the guided autobiography group experience.

Music

It is gratifying to see the looks of recognition and excitement when group members are greeted by music from their past. You can maximize this response by choosing music from specific periods. For example, generally, the music that is most salient for people is the music they listened to when they were adolescents and young adults. By targeting these periods, you can stimulate recall and greatly enhance the sensitization process.

Music can also be combined with recall of major historical events for a particular age group. For example, you might play a popular tune from 1945 and ask members to share what they were doing when they heard the news that victory had been won in Europe during World War II.

Similarly, you might ask group members to bring in their favorite recordings from the past. This not only stimulates recall but provides an opportunity for sharing the memories associated with the music, for example, how their parents reacted to the music, where they listened to it, and who their friends were who liked the same music.

Music also might be used to reflect the diverse backgrounds of group members. To accomplish this, you might request that members bring in recordings that best reflect their particular cohort or that are an important part of their ethnic, regional, or family identities.

Food

In Chapter 2 we discussed the use of food to encourage participation in the guided autobiography group. As a shared responsibility, bringing snacks can be a technique to encourage discussion of food as an aspect of each other's heritage. Like music, foods can bring to mind memories that are otherwise forgotten and enhance recall of experiences from the past.

Fragrances

The leader can bring in sample fragrances to be passed around in the group. Group members might then be asked what, if any, memories the fragrances brought to mind. Some examples of fragrances that have been used in past groups are

fresh-cut grass
fall leaves
hay
baby or dusting powder
cinnamon
candle smoke
dittographic paper
fresh-printed pages of a book
finger paints

suntan lotion
rubbing alcohol
unshelled peanuts
pine needles
spices
incense

The Use of Puppets

Puppets are sometimes used to encourage people to distance them-selves from the disclosure of experiences and feelings that are difficult to express directly or openly. Although guided autobiography is not therapy, the theory behind the use of puppets in therapy can be applied to it.

Puppet shows can be organized in conjunction with guided autobiog-raphy or independently as a separate kind of experience in autobiography. Two or three members of the group can safely speak through hand pup-pets of feelings that might be difficult to express in the first person. The moving mouth of a hand puppet held at arm's length may provide a secu-rity of distance to tell the important life story one step removed. A Japa-nese psychologist, Tachibana, in a personal communication, once spoke to the authors about indirection dealing with life story. He said, "One may allude to things in the heart without speaking directly of them."

Whether actual puppets are brought into the group, or people are en-couraged to "speak" through their hands as imaginary characters, this technique is useful in fostering freedom of expression. If employed in an atmosphere of relaxation and enjoyment, the use of puppets can be both fun and comical and can release old memories and feelings.

Chapter *7*

Mastering Potential Obstacles in the Group Process

PROBLEMS may arise in conducting guided autobiography groups, ranging from a specific group member's insensitive behavior to lack of support from the institutional setting. There are many ways to manage these problems, and the best will be based on your own judgment of the situation and your personal style. It is important to recognize the early warning signs of such problems. Difficulties in interpersonal relations and institutional adjustments tend to arise during the first two sessions when uncertainty is highest and relationships have not yet formed. For this reason, we have to move quickly to resolve problems early in the process. In this chapter we review the warning signs related to common concerns and discuss successful techniques to manage them.

Overenrollment

A seemingly positive problem is overenrollment, that is, many more people than anticipated respond to the initial invitation to join a guided autobiography group. This is a sign that the guided autobiography process has been publicized or "marketed" well and that you have successfully motivated your target group. Overenrollment, however, can present a major obstacle to the acceptance of future programs if less-than-careful planning leads to a disappointed community.

No group member will benefit from guided autobiography if there is an atmosphere of competition for time or, worse yet, if there is chaos. Being listened to is as important to every member as having the opportunity to review one's life stories. As the group leader, you must guard against overenrollment which might result in insufficient time and attention. Misdirected kindness in allowing extra enrollees, or last minute sign-ups who "just got the word," can mar a group experience.

One way to avoid this problem is to invite interest but specify that a limited number can be accepted. Those people to be included in this number might be personally chosen by you in accordance with your goals for the group (e.g., new residents of a nursing home) and the recommendations outlined in Chapter 2. Or, you might simply offer enrollment on a first-come, first-served basis. Ideally, those who can not participate at the present time could be offered the opportunity to participate in a future group.

In large settings, where such problems might be anticipated, the authors recommend developing a network of potential group leaders. As noted earlier, we have conducted as many as six groups simultaneously with the use of multiple leaders. We try to anticipate the enrollment and to confirm arrangements with the appropriate number of leaders; at the same time we make tentative agreements with other leaders who stand by to lead groups should last-minute overenrollment occur. The likelihood of overenrollment varies with the setting (for example, university, community college, senior center, or nursing home) and the degree of control the leader has over participation.

Counterproductive Group Members

Problems with specific group members arise when someone in the group has poor interpersonal skills, suffers from a severe need for attention, or is misplaced in the group due to cognitive or emotional disability.

Wherever possible, it is helpful for you to meet individually with all group members prior to their entrance into the group. This will provide an opportunity to identify those who may have personal styles that would be counterproductive to the group process and to limit or dissuade such members from entering the group before the first meeting. This can best be done by directing these persons to other groups or individual therapy that might be better suited to their needs.

To assist you in recognizing potential problem members, we have developed the following list of prototypic characters who seem to appear fairly regularly in group meetings: (1) the monopolizer, (2) the career group member, (3) the amateur therapist, and (4) the nonparticipant.

The Monopolizer

Appearing in many books on group processes and techniques, this member presents him- or herself almost invariably to participate in group experiences. In need of great amounts of attention and primarily interested in being listened to, monopolizers consistently run over the time allotted for their stories and have an incredible talent for drawing attention to their own lives even when the focus is someone else's story. They may use every opportunity to "relate to" the other members, but you may soon notice leaps into disconnected content areas that focus attention on themselves. They may become visibly impatient when others are speaking and may thwart your attempts to redirect attention away from them.

Monopolizers can seriously disrupt the guided autobiography group process. They require much attention from the group leader. As frustrating as this member may be, it is important to protect the group process. This can often be accomplished by offering the monopolizer an opportunity to meet with you once outside the group to discuss what he or she may do beyond the guided autobiography process to expand on the life story and share it with others, such as family members (see Chapter 8). Or, it can be accomplished by validating the monopolizer's contribution to the group but firmly redirecting attention to other members. This is demonstrated in the following example:

> Group Member 1 has just completed the story of his career development. Once having been a priest, he left the church during the 1960s to join the Peace Corps and later returned to school to become a social worker.
>
> The Monopolizer: It must have been a hard decision to leave the priesthood. How did your family react? I converted to Christianity early in my marriage, and it took years for my relationship with my parents to return to normal.
>
> Note that this would be a good example of the developmental exchange if the Monopolizer stopped at this point and allowed Group Member 1 to respond to the question of how his family reacted. Less interested in the answer to his question, however, and having earlier continued speaking beyond the time allotted for sharing his own story, the Monopolizer went on to detail the history of his relationship with his mother.
>
> The Monopolizer: It's not that my mother and I were ever very close, but it was even harder after my conversion. I think that she

had a hard time accepting the fact that she never had a daughter. Being the only son, I . . .

Group Leader: Our family history often plays a role in other areas of our lives. What you're saying is very interesting and I hope we hear more about it in one of your stories. But, I'm intrigued by your original question, so right now let's return to John (Group Member 1). John, how did your family react?

In this example, the group leader validated the contribution of the monopolizer by requesting that he continue his story at some other time and by using his own question to redirect the focus to the original member. The message was clear that this was not the time for the monopolizer to tell his own story, but it also reinforced the monopolizer for relevant questions that focus on other members' stories.

You must be firm in communicating that the group experience requires shared time and focus, both in the group and during your individual interactions with monopolizers. It is important to remember, however, that this norm is most likely to be accepted by the monopolizer if the person feels there will be additional opportunities to be heard in the future.

The Career Group Member

Some people engage in group experiences on a constant basis. This can be valuable, particularly for older adults who have retired and may have limited social networks. What distinguishes the "career" group member, however, is that this person views him- or herself as an expert on group experiences. This person may disrupt the current group process by frequent references to and comparisons with past groups he or she has participated in. Such comparisons can be particularly disconcerting for the group leader if they are used to challenge the methods and conduct of the guided autobiography group.

These members are best dealt with as early and as frankly as possible. Simply note that the guided autobiography group *is* different from other groups, but urge that the focus be maintaind on *the guided autobiography* process. It is useful to acknowledge the person's wealth of experience in group processes and to invite patience with the new experience until after the last class. You could note that any insights into how the guided autobiography group might be enhanced would be welcomed at that point.

The Amateur Therapist

Related to the career group member, amateur therapists feel that past experiences in therapy groups or their own insights have afforded them a unique ability to interpret other persons' lives and behavior. They may participate in the guided autobiography process more because of a desire to play therapist with others' stories than from a desire to review their own life stories. Such a member may be particularly problematic if "insights" tend to be personal judgments regarding the mental or emotional stability of other members. This kind of judgment often involves interpretation of another member's behavior or feelings as either normal or abnormal.

To manage the amateur therapist in the group, it is necessary to emphasize strongly the group norm of nonjudgmentalism. In rare instances, it may be necessary to do so on an individual basis; however, wherever possible, it is best to avoid direct criticism of any member's behavior in the group. Subtle contradiction that pointedly reinforces nonjudgmental behavior can be used (1) to protect the member being analyzed by the amateur therapist and (2) to deter future analysis or judgment. The scenario below demonstrates this technique.

> Member 1: Since my mother's death, I never go to funerals. I just don't feel comfortable grieving openly.
>
> Member 2 (Amateur Therapist): It sounds to me more like you are avoiding the whole issue of death. You need to face it head on.
>
> Group Leader: So, in the group we have people who grieve in different ways. This is not unusual. Some cultures don't have funerals at all as we know them. I think that it's important to recognize that not everyone responds just as we do—there is no right or wrong way to deal with the loss of a loved one.

The Nonparticipant

The nonparticipant can take a number of forms, for the most part distinguished by degree of silence.

Rarely, someone may join the group, insist that he or she would like to attend each meeting, but consistently "forget" or "not have the time" to write the autobiographical story assignments. Or, a member may refuse to share his or her stories with the group. These members are very disruptive to the group process and should be referred to a different kind of group experience early on.

Other members may read their two-page autobiographical stories but withhold any emotional information. This represents a challenge to the developmental exchange. In some instances, a person needs the door to be opened. Most important may be a sign that his or her feelings are meaningful to the group and, especially, the group leader. A simple question, such as "How did that make you feel," can often release the tension surrounding emotional expression.

In other instances, a member may not feel comfortable openly expressing emotion, despite your welcoming of such expression. As long as this person is not obstructing others, he or she is best left to harvest those aspects of the guided autobiography process with which he or she feels comfortable.

Frequently, members may decline to share one or two of their autobiographical stories with the group. Often, this arises in connection with a theme that is highly emotional for the particular member involved. The leader might suggest that the member write the story for his or her own use and only share it later on if he or she feels comfortable. It is also helpful to stress that not all the written information needs to be shared with the group. Although the leader will have to intervene if a given member is disrupting the group process by refusing to share the majority of autobiographical stories, there is no reason that a member should be forced to read every story. Since this is not therapy, it is important not to invade highly guarded emotional territory.

Signs of Depression and What to Do

Persons who are clinically depressed should be referred to a mental health facility or licensed therapist for professional assistance. Ideally, referral should occur at the first contact, whether through written materials, staff opinion, or an initial conversation. Persons needing referral should not be included in the guided autobiography group.

In our many years of experience, we have not had a group member report having become depressed as a result of the guided autobiography group. This may be related to research findings that demonstrate that dissatisfied persons (Coleman, 1974, 1986) and depressed persons (McMahon and Rhudick, 1967) are less likely to reminisce than nondepressed or satisfied persons. Thus, those suffering from depression or severe dissatisfaction are not likely to present themselves for the guided autobiography process. In support of the potential benefits of the process, research conducted at the University of Southern California in the senior author's laboratory has compared guided autobiography group members before and after engaging in the process and has demonstrated either improved affect or no change.

There is some evidence in the research literature on life-review techniques that life review may trigger a depressive response. However, it is important to examine this response in the context in which it was elicited. In reviewing the literature, we discovered that many of the persons studied had presented themselves for treatment at a mental health facility, had engaged in life review, and were then diagnosed as depressed. Here one should ask why the persons had come to the mental health facility in the first place. Similarly, in a case study cited by Shute (1986), in his cautionary note on life review, the individual in the case described was referred to a community mental health center because of a noticeable disengagement from usual activities, a known signal of the onset of depression. Clearly, there was some indication of potential depression before life review.

Regardless, the responsible group leader will seek to properly refer persons who are depressed before their engaging in the group and will monitor group members' responses during the process to ensure that any member who is in need of professional counseling is appropriately referred (see below).

Older adults may be particularly vulnerable to depression due to the increased likelihood of significant losses in later life. Death of a spouse, sibling, or friend, or unwanted life changes associated with disability and retirement, may lead to depression. Particularly if you are aware of recent losses of this nature, it is important to guard for depression among group members. Mood changes are a natural part of life at any age. Sad memories may evoke feelings of regret or temporary melancholy. It is also natural, however, for such sadness to lift and for pleasant memories or simply a new day to return us to a more happy mood. Depression is signalled if a person does not improve in affect or if melancholy increases over time.

The following warning signs are proposed by Bumagin and Hirn (1990) to identify depression:

- Notable decreases in the speed of response, particularly a slowing in speech patterns
- Notable decreases or increases in sleep
- Recent loss of interest in food or the beginning of overeating
- Self-neglect, often signalled by notable changes in physical appearance
- Increased agitation

- Confusion
- Hostility
- Suicidal thoughts

To these might be added:

- A strong emphasis on feelings of helplessness in a person's autobiographical stories
- Highly recurrent, or especially unexplained, crying in the group
- Uncharacteristic withdrawal from social interaction
- Singular focus on losses and feelings of despair throughout autobiographical stories

Persons who demonstrate such behaviors should be referred to a professional counselor with whom they can discuss and, hopefully, work through their feelings of despair and hopelessness. Family or institutional caregivers should be made aware of the group leader's observations and the referral advised.

Where a caregiver is involved, meet with this person before the older adult's entrance into the guided autobiography group. Make it clear that this is not therapy and that no profound behavioral or emotional change should be expected. If the caregivers are seeking therapeutic treatment for the older adult, they should be referred elsewhere.

Ensuring Institutional Support

The success of the guided autobiography group depends in part on the commitment and support of the institution in which it is conducted. Particularly in sites such as nursing homes, the cooperation of the administrative staff and caregivers is essential to ensure that group members are able to attend each session and that there is positive reinforcement for continued participation in the group. Without this support, group members may feel that they are forced to choose between activities or that their relationship with staff will be harmed by participation in the guided autobiography group.

In most cases, such support comes easily. Generally, families and personnel of senior care facilities are enthusiastic about the potentials of guided autobiography and welcome the availability of such groups. In some instances, however, staff members may be wary of new or outside members. The key to engaging their support is enlisting the cooperation and support of the top administrator and, where applicable, the head of nursing. These people will greatly influence the degree of cooperation provided by direct-care providers. Without this cooperation, difficulties may arise, such as:

- Group members not being up and dressed to attend the group meetings on time
- Group members being scheduled for conflicting appointments, such as physical therapy or doctor visits
- Inconsistency in scheduling of rooms, such that the group is shuffled around from meeting to meeting or forced to meet in a room in which other activities are occurring simultaneously
- Lack of cooperation in preparing the room for the group, for example, insufficient seating or difficult access
- Group members being required to leave early due to scheduling conflicts
- Member attrition resulting from negative reactions on the part of the staff
- Staff members' failing to inform group leaders of pertinent information about group members, such as signs of depressive behavior or decreased cognitive capacity
- The role of the group leader being sabotaged because of staff criticism

You can employ a number of strategies to ensure cooperation and to develop lasting rapport with key personnel and staff. Initial interactions are particularly important and should be carefully planned. The following is a list of initial steps and strategies for developing a positive working relationship in long-term care facilities and nursing homes. These strategies can easily be adapted to other sites, such as senior centers, where the staff titles may differ but roles are similar with regard to the ability of group members to benefit as much as possible from the guided autobiography process.

1. First meet with the senior administrator to propose and outline the progression of the guided autobiography group process. It will help to review what you hope to accomplish and to specify the anticipated benefits for group members.
2. Seek the administrator's input regarding key staff to be recruited to facilitate the logistical arrangements for the group, and engage his or her cooperation in creating a positive relationship with this staff, for example, the director of nursing.

3. Develop a rapport with the nurses and nurses' aides who assist group members in preparing for the group. In noninstitutional settings, develop a rapport with family members and other caregivers who may be responsible for providing transportation and other support. It is helpful to learn names, to show appreciation for efforts to make group members available, and to provide some feedback regarding observations you have made about the impact of the group on the specific patient or family member.

4. Whenever possible, meet with administrators and staff before beginning the group to explain the guided autobiography process, its benefits, and the importance of attending all the meetings on time and for the complete time allotted.

5. Gently remind the staff about meetings in advance, and set a predictable schedule that will not conflict with other activities in the facility.

6. Welcome feedback, including criticism; listen carefully to all comments; and wherever appropriate provide feedback on what actions have been taken.

7. Carefully plan the group experience. Arrive early to check on the room, assist in the set-up, and so on. Let the staff know you are willing to help as needed with the preparation for the group.

Most problems with institutional support arise because of insufficient or poor communication. These seven strategies will help to avoid difficulties and to ensure support both for the leader and for those who wish to participate as members.

Chapter 8

The Next Steps after Guided Autobiography

SOME GROUP MEMBERS may have the impression that after having done a guided autobiography there will be nothing else to do. The last word will have been spoken. While completing a guided autobiography may result in a written life story to be copied for friends and relations, it need not be an end. The first trip through one's autobiography is often a process of collecting ideas, memories, and materials, and of increasing sensitization to the major issues of life. It is worthwhile to go through it a second time to elaborate on details and examine the same life story from an expanded, more enlightened perspective.

The senior author of this book was once asked by Dr. Robert Butler to do an extensive life interview with Dr. Charlotte Buhler, a distinguished psychologist and former resident of Los Angeles. Butler requested that Buhler be brought through her life history two times. She and the senior author spent about three two-hour interview sessions, beginning with the early part of her life and going through to the present in the first session and then repeating the process in the second and third sessions. It was surprising how many more details she recalled on the second trip through her life history.

In the interval between a first and second autobiographical review, there is time to review family documents, look up old photographs and correspondence, and talk to relatives and long-time friends. The second time through one's autobiography can be travelled with the same group, with the intention of keeping one's motivation up by participating in the group process and perhaps preparing more systematic, comprehensive material for eventual formal or informal publication. We have had a number of people participate in the guided autobiography process two times, separated by several years. If all members of a group are "second timers," the format can be changed to include more examples of autobiographies, to provide the participants with alternatives. Photocopying and desktop publishing now permit the preparation of small numbers of copies at a reasonable cost. Copies of old photographs can also be prepared for inclusion in a text.

The group leader may anticipate conducting guided autobiography I (GA I) and guided autobiography II (GA II), the latter being primarily for more serious persons who want to do a publishable or near-publishable account of their lives for circulation in a family. The group leader can judge the seriousness of the intent to write and review the life and can evaluate trade-offs between maintaining the continuity of one group and incorporating new members. Carryover friendships are of value in terms of support. At the same time, however, there is a trade-off between the support of established relationships and the motivational value derived from a change in membership between GA I and GA II.

The leader will observe with experience that he or she will become the repository of many autobiographies, including those that are finished after completing GA I. That is, many persons will feel they have had enough experience with the first course to then, in the privacy of their own homes, do a more systematic job of writing the stories of their lives. Despite their individual effort, the first group tends to be their reference group, and they will look to the leader for acceptance. They will likely want to give the leader a copy as a gift and perhaps for comment.

A Continuous Search for Meaning

The writer of a guided autobiography usually has several motives for doing it. One motive is the personal search for meaning in life; another is to put together a legacy for others. Probably, the search for meaning is the basic motive from which the leaving of a legacy derives. We have to have attachments, and other people must have meaning in our lives for us to want to give them our guided autobiography.

Salvatore Maddi (1970, p. 137) wrote: "If a person works, raises a family, joins clubs, gives parties, falls in love, or meets challenges, it is because these are the activities that have somehow achieved meaning for him." Writing one's autobiography is perhaps the most manifest search for meaning in comparison with the more indirect or mini-searches we do each day. The first trip through guided autobiography is not the end of the search for meaning but rather a starting point.

An inability to find meaning in the activities and experiences of a long life is a bleak prospect, one that is forestalled by a trip through life, a review of major branching points. Just as a second nature hike in the same woods will tend to turn up more birds and plants, a second autobiographical review will turn up more details of events and relationships, helping to meet the late-life need for increased meaning and integration.

In preparation for GA II or for a personal review, interviews can be set up with relatives and friends following GA I. These can be generally exploratory or focused on a particular period or event, as illustrated in the following example:

> When Jim's mother was in her eighties, he had the chance to talk with her about the first place he lived after his birth. She told him how he climbed off the back porch after a gate had been installed. This interaction reminded him of more details about where he lived and where he had played with other children. What came out of the conversation was a view of himself as a more exploratory, "hard to keep out of mischief" boy than his earlier image. This led him, when he later went back to Chicago, to take some pictures of places he had lived. Should he now want to leave his life story to others, he has more details and pictures to include. Both his view of himself and his autobiographical document were enlarged.

Aunts, uncles, cousins, and old family friends are watching you grow up and live your life. They will have some interesting stories about how the family functioned and how you fit into the family. They may have some photos of old family events you never saw or had forgotten. Old photos can be easily copied.

> A relative told Jim that his parents bought a house in Chicago two years before he was born. The house was built by his grandfather, who sold it to Jim's parents for $400. The house was next door to the grandparents, which proved to be too close for Jim's mother's comfort. Jim never knew this family background until he talked to other family members. Yet, it shed much light on the history of relationships in his family.

Other family members may have family trees they can share with you along with pictures of family reunions. Your first effort in guided autobiography may serve as a catalyst to motivate you to seek this material.

High school and college reunions are excellent sources for additional material for a second trip through guided autobiography. Use a tape recorder and get the information from other persons. Do not be surprised, however, if other persons' recollections are not the same as yours. Most likely, their memories will add information you never knew. Talking about teachers, basketball games, dances, dates, and where you ate lunch will evoke rich material for later review, as can be seen in the following example:

> Jim's fiftieth high school reunion gave him contacts that are now maintained by mail. One man loaned Jim his high school annual, since Jim had lost his during an early move. The annual was a gold mine of names and events. Some high school friends had moved to Jim's area, and conversations resulted about who took whom to the senior prom. He was very surprised at some of the things that had happened over fifty years ago, things that had influenced his life but about which he was unaware.

In addition to visiting people from your past, you can add questions to your holiday greeting cards and ask about the past, to fill gaps about your growing up. Important places from your past can also be revisited.

> John was a navigator on a Blenheim Bomber when it was shot down over Belgium during the early days of World War II. He was found unconscious in the plane after it crashed in a farmer's field, and he was taken to a nearby village to be nursed by a young woman. Forty years later, the Belgium town had a celebration to which John was invited. He then met the now elderly woman who had nursed him after the crash. She told him details he had never known of the crash, his rescue, and his injuries. All this now had an important place in his personal history documents and was reflected in his guided autobiography.
>
> For John, the visit to Belgium filled in the gap on some important details of his life. It was also apparent in his life-story essays that there had been an incubation process for many years. He had a curiosity about what happened in the air over Belgium and his rescue that never reached a focus until he retired and had the time to think about it. He was then motivated to make the trip to Belgium for information gathering in the form of an anniversary celebration.

The group leader in GA II can help members of the group plan and conduct searches for more documentation of their growing up and growing old. Other members of the group can help by describing their successes in finding information. Discussions will help to form a strategic approach for securing more documentation. Later life and retirement can unexpectedly bring to awareness things that were important but put out of mind "until you got around to it." There are gaps in our memories that apparently create tensions, and the memories surface when the saliency increases to the level where it breaks into our consciousness. Life is a search for meaning, and guided autobiography is a way of making it more effective.

Exploring Publishing Interest and Potential

In GA II, the strongly motivated may want to consider publishing their polished life stories. This can be done at several levels: securing a commercial publisher, finding a vanity press in which the individual will underwrite the costs, or producing your story with a personal computer and a word-processing or desktop-publishing program. The last is inexpensive and may lend itself to doing a limited number of copies for family members and friends. On the other hand, a typewritten or handwritten document is simple and it can be photocopied, and it may meet the individual's needs.

For those who want to explore more formal publication, additional time should be spent reading autobiographies and criticizing their content and format in a group. Reading other autobiographies sharpens our power of appraisal of our own work. What makes a book publishable and a commercial success is not always that its author is a popular public figure. The story has to be intrinsically interesting. Simple people often have powerful stories to tell, but judgment about the potential interest is a matter for skilled editors.

Most members of a guided autobiography group will not want to put the necessary effort into preparing a polished document for publication. For this reason, the few who want to go further with publication might be encouraged to join a writing group with professional writing interests as the primary focus.

Other Writing Experiences

The primary emphasis in this book is the enhancement of the search for meaning in life, with a secondary emphasis on leaving a legacy to others. Little emphasis is given to publication, since this is not the primary purpose for most participants. In GA II the next steps can be taken to enlarge the scope of one's search for meaning in becoming sensitized to old memories and different points of view.

Creative Writing

In GA II a group leader can have members write additional autobiographical poems. They can be asked to write a poem about their childhood in the first, second, or third person. Productive assignments can be made from such topics as starting school, first birthdays, or family thanksgivings. Members might try to write a poem about "the search for me" or "where to find me." (For more on this topic, see Chapter 6.) As the group members write, hear, and read each other's poems, they become more confident with subjective interpretations and alternative points of view.

Short essays can also be undertaken in GA II. These can be oriented around the history of a school, business, community, or church but written in the first person as the observer. These autobiographical essays can find a place in present-day newsletters, alumni magazines, local newspapers, or magazines of national organizations. Anniversary dates of organizations bring out calls for material about the "early days." Writing these essays improves writing skills and sharpens the focus on the past. An essential element in the process is reading them aloud to a group for comments and suggestions for revision. This process is one of becoming more sensitive to the material but also less sensitive to criticism of the writing itself.

Writing a Journal

As we have discussed throughout this book, life histories are written for many purposes, and they may take many forms, with different emphases on content. A biography is a written account of a person's life by another person. Reading biographies can sensitize and open one's perspective on life experiences that might be vicariously shared with the protagonist. Autobiographical accounts are of one's own life and can range from the total sweep of a life from its beginning until the moment of writing, to a focus on a small vignette, a day, or part of a day. To prepare for doing one's autobiography, or as part of GA II, diaries or journals may be kept that are autobiographical and give a daily record of events, experiences, and observations.

The focus of the autobiographical content is the experience of the individual and the individual's interpretation of events. It is an inside picture of a life as it has been lived. In contrast, biographies interpret a life from an external perspective. A joint perspective arises in the recording of oral history, in which the individual is used as an avenue to the interpretation of an historical event or period. Oral history seeks to reconstruct the event, the context of the experience, and is less concerned than other historical methods about how the event fits into other events that occurred before and after. Similarly, it is less concerned with the inner person than is biography or autobiography. Thus, the oral history of World War I or the Great Depression will attempt to recover the details of those times by using the individual's recollections as the source; it does not attempt to reconstruct the individual's life.

Some individuals keep diaries and journals with the thought that one day they will write a comprehensive autobiography. In writing the autobiography, most single days are omitted because there were no turning points, important interactions, insights, or accidents that helped to form the life in a major way. There is a common thread in a diary, a journal, and an autobiography, that is, the focus on the individual's interpretation of the experiences of a life.

Progoff (1975) described the keeping of intensive journals as a process for reconstructing the flow of life. It, like autobiography, does not attempt to put an external or theoretical framework upon life, but it, too, can change the flow of a life. Progoff says that the intensive journal is "*beyond psychotherapy* because it takes a *transpsychological* approach to what had been thought of as psychological problems. Here the word *transpsychological* means that it brings about therapeutic effects, not by striving towards therapy, but by providing active techniques that enable an individual to draw upon his inherent resources or becoming a whole person" (Progoff, 1975, p. 9). For these reasons, journal writing can be a powerful addition to guided autobiography, helping to inform the autobiography and to motivate continued introspection beyond the group process.

Autobiographical methods are designed to heighten the interpretation and insights an individual may have in his or her life. In addition to questions that explore how the life has flowed and what forces have shaped it, there is the question: How do *most* people's lives flow? Runyan (1984) distinguishes between the life history of an individual as a *method* for having the respondent recount the story of his or her life, and the life history as a *subject matter* that provides insights for developing generalizations about individuals' lives. He posits that there are three different levels of life stories in terms of generalities: (1) whether the life story is true of all persons, (2) whether it is true of a group of persons (e.g., sex, race, or culture), and (3) whether it is true only of particular human beings. Guided autobiography, the intensive journal technique developed by Progoff, and other written methods of personal introspection are designed to heighten the recall of memories. The choice is whether one moves from the broad to specific, or the specific to the broad. For the individual, it is understanding of the self that is sought. In developing a legacy, it may be important also to focus on what applies more broadly to the group (e.g., family, culture) and, possibly, to all persons. A journal is an excellent arena in which to explore these different aspects of one's life experiences.

The foregoing is not unlike the issue of whether one should describe a forest by starting with a leaf on an individual tree and then moving to a broader perspective, or by beginning with a distant view of the forest and ending up with the fluttering of an individual leaf. Obviously, we favor beginning with a guided look of the forest, in which likely clusters of experience are pointed out for examination. Clearly, if one is going to describe the fabric of one's life, one needs both warp and woof—threads travelling longitudinally as well as crosswise—with individual strands forming the base on which patterns evolve and form a dynamic picture, as in a tapestry.

Keeping a diary or a journal, just as engaging in guided autobiography in a small group, may not be to everyone's liking or disposition. The thesis here, however, as in Progoff's method, is that there is a great benefit to be derived from constructing the tapestry of one's life.

Creating a Legacy

There is a feeling of permanence about being recorded in a book, not only for the writer but for others as well. How we see our lives and the lives of others recorded is a matter of active interest, as is a concern about how the facts are represented or misrepresented. To some extent all of us want attention from others, and one pathway into others' awareness is the writing of our life story. Our quests for attention and perpetuity are in part expressed in passing on our life stories to heirs we may never see. In China, Korea, and Japan there is a tradition of family books in which all members are recorded. Family members of thirty generations ago are duly registered, and the book is passed into the safekeeping of the oldest son. For example:

A Korean professor who took our course in guided autobiography indicated that a main element in his identity was his role as the oldest son. When he returned to Korea he was to have the responsibility for the family book that had twenty-seven generations recorded in it. When we remarked that this was a great many, he replied that it was not so many, "some Chinese families have even longer recorded family histories."

In the West, the tradition of the passed-on family Bible provided a perpetual thread with the past. This tradition is fading, but perhaps in the post-industrial society there will be the time and skills to write autobiographies that may replace the family Bible and help our successors answer questions about who they are and where they came from. This would seem a healthy pursuit and one that might help to relieve some of the "existential sickness" found in our high-speed society where there is little time to find out who we are.

The birth of a grandchild may stimulate the writing of the legacy. Also, a family reunion may provide the opportunity to pass on to others copies of their history as interpreted by one member. Furthermore, the reunion celebration can motivate other family members to write. Those who lead autobiography groups may find it useful to point out that the family reunion can be an occasion to celebrate a life story and a common legacy.

Guided Autobiography and Medusa's Head

In Greek mythology, Medusa was one of three horrible creatures whose hair consisted of writhing snakes. Anyone who looked directly at Medusa's head turned into stone. The hero Perseus was able to avoid turning to stone and to cut off the head of Medusa by looking at her reflection in his shining shield. This myth is adaptable to describe our attempts to deal with some painful memories in our past. We may be so afraid to look at some memories directly that we become paralyzed with fear or "turn to stone."

Painful recollections are often put out of mind because they are too difficult to face head on. The fear of facing a Medusa, the memory of a traumatic event, leads to denial or repression of the anxiety-laden memory. The memory may not only be put out of mind, it may be repressed and actively put out of the reach of recall.

One of the principles of psychotherapy is that a repressed memory may lead to strange twists in behavior or to disturbing contradictions in our behavior, in addition to creating mental blind spots for the events themselves.

A participant, in retelling her life story, her guided autobiography, may stumble onto a walled-off memory. This may be accompanied by insight, or the "aha experience," but also by unnerving feelings of anxiety. The security offered by the group is reassuring and reduces anxiety such that the individual feels strong enough to risk recalling a walled-off or entombed memory. There is no intent in the guided autobiography process to deliberately exhume repressed memories, but we sometimes get a reflected point of view of a lurking Medusa's head in the shield of another group member. Sometimes we feel strong enough that we encourage indirect recall, face indirectly a frightful figure and cut off its head, since we are no longer afraid of turning to stone.

In a book about writing life stories, Bernard Selling (1989) discussed writing about the inner you. He noted that psychotherapists spend a great deal of time helping people "get in touch with themselves, meaning, in part, developing the capacity to become aware of their feelings" (p. 60). Many of us have become emotionally blind to events of our development and have to put special effort into recovering a clear view of our inner self.

For some curious and motivated persons there is an urge to explore the inner self, but the difficulty of this process necessitates more than one journey through guided autobiography. Through continued explorations of the inner self, the confident and curious among us can uncover old memories and feelings of the past that left their mark on us, marks we often do not wish to note.

After guided autobiography, a person may join a creative writing group to write indirectly about his or her inner self through fiction and poetry or even drama. The energy involved in old feelings makes much, perhaps most, writing, whether intended or not, autobiographical. Selling notes, "The ability to transfer these feelings onto paper is what makes us writers" (1989, p. 60).

For some persons, creative life-story writing may be a useful next step after guided autobiography. Through it they may overcome their fear of writing and may experience revitalization. In conducting classes on life-story writing, Selling noted that the process of writing was immensely therapeutic for each person. He also pointed out that there is a therapeutic as well as informative outcome of being congratulated by class members for your work.

If we look at a repressed memory directly, we feel we will turn to stone, that is, die. Sometimes the contents of the withheld past spill out seemingly by chance. Guided autobiography is not intended to draw out deliberately the painfully hidden past. Another approach to the life story is to proceed totally by indirection, looking at the life from a more objective vantage point, of which writing drama or participating in story telling may be a vitalizing influence. Further insight can be provided by indirection, by participating in other writing experiences after guided autobiography.

Chapter 9

A Professional's Guide to the Literature, and Implications for Future Research

THIS LAST CHAPTER is written for professionals and graduate students interested in the theoretical underpinnings that spawned the development of the guided autobiography process. It is written also to provide those interested in research on autobiography with a professional's guide to the current literature; that is, it is an overview of current thoughts regarding why people write their autobiographies and of the status of research that utilizes autobiographies as a source of data to explore issues of personal development and sociological and historical influences.

Due to space limitations, this chapter is not intended as a thorough review of the literature. Rather, it is designed to provide the reader with enough material to form an understanding and to stimulate future exploration.

We believe that this is a vital area of research and scholarship, in need of further study and future research leaders. For too many years, personal accounts either have been given cursory treatment or have been ignored in research designed to increase understanding of individuals and the human condition. Those scientists who have developed cogent methods for accessing and analyzing these powerful data are to be congratulated. We hope that future research leaders will follow in their stead. With this as our motive, we have included materials designed to orient and stimulate graduate students and others to conduct research in this important area.

Who Writes Autobiographies?

In this section, we will provide an overview of research on the history of the written autobiography and explore autobiographical endeavors that might be missed by current research due to methodological constraints and biases that discount anecdotal accounts. It is important to begin with a definition of terms. Here, the term *autobiography* refers to a written personal account of an individual's life story. *Life review* denotes the purposeful recollection of the events and emotions of one's life story, not necessarily in written form. *Reminiscence* is the recalling of past events or feelings and does not denote any specific purpose or attempt to be inclusive or thorough with regard to the life course.

Historical Documents

The first record of a written autobiography dates back as early as 400 A.D. to St. Augustine's *Confessions,* although some researchers (e.g., Lejeune, 1986; Roos, 1988) suggest that the fragments of even earlier efforts can be found in the archives of Mesopotamia, Egypt, India, and China.

The early autobiographies of record were generally written as "confessions" or "memoirs," mostly by clergy or philosophers. Writing one's autobiographical account was uncommon in early times, primarily due to high levels of illiteracy in early societies and a devaluation of introspection by the "common man" (Weintraub, 1978).

The Renaissance brought with it an increased sense of the importance of individuals, and written autobiographies became more common. During the seventeenth century, English became a written language and increases in the numbers of autobiographies continued. Such increases were particularly reflected in societies undergoing radical social changes, which included England (Olney, 1980). This trend continued through the eighteenth and nineteenth centuries, with autobiographies often written as commentaries by those seeking social transformation (for examples of such works, see Wachter, 1988).

In the last two centuries, the advent of public education, coupled with greater acceptance of the individual as a potent force in society, has led to an expansion of published autobiographical accounts to include ones written by persons from many walks of life, for example, politicians, educators, criminals, and business people.

Although the practice of writing one's autobiography has gained broader acceptance over time, there still appear to be some general characteristics that determine who writes their autobiographies. For example, an autobiography is more likely to emerge if the person is introspective or self-reflective, is self-confident and has positive self-regard, and has some belief in his or her own uniqueness (Wrightsman, 1988).

Age has also been found to be a predictor of who will write his or her autobiography, with autobiographies often written by those who perceive themselves as near the end of their lives or as representing a bygone era. Older adults have been found to be more past-oriented and more likely to engage in autobiographical memory in response to the use of prompt-words (Sperbeck, Whitbourne, and Hoyer, 1986). Older adults are also more likely to be introspective, focusing on the inner self rather than the outer conditions of life (Birren, in press). Such introspection leads a person to engage in life review as new actions are reviewed in the context of what has gone before.

In addition to these personal characteristics, there appears to be some correlation between one's occupation and autobiographical writing. For example, few autobiographies have been written by people whose careers are in business or farming, while numerous examples exist for those in the fields of communication, entertainment, medicine, research, and political science (Wrightsman, 1988). Such distinctions, however, appear to be diminishing as popular culture, and particularly television, produces "media personalities" from a wide variety of settings. Notable examples of this new trend are the multiple best-selling autobiographies of Lee Iacocca, the chief executive officer of a major automobile-manufacturing corporation.

Finally, there appears to be a motivation for writing one's autobiography for public consumption. Clark (1935, as cited in Wrightsman) classified these motives into four categories:

1. Appeal for sympathy
2. Need for self-justification
3. Desire for appreciation and praise
4. Need for artistic communication

Allport (1942), on the other hand, distinguished as many as twelve motives for writing one's autobiography:

1. Special pleading to prove one is more sinned against than sinning
2. Exhibitionism
3. Desire for order in one's life
4. Literary delight (aesthetic pleasure of writing)
5. Securing a personal perspective

6. Relief from tension
7. Redemption and social reincorporation
8. Monetary gain
9. Fulfillment of an assignment, such as for a class or admission to a particular school or program
10. Assistance in therapy
11. Scientific interest
12. Public service and example

In contemporary society, the role of the publisher as acquisition editor should not be overlooked; many publishers employ individuals who solicit, and may play a role in developing manuscripts for which a market has been identified. As Allport indicates, monetary gain is a key factor in some persons' decisions to write their autobiographies. Since in contemporary society there is a strong market for autobiographies written by those in the public eye, publishers play a role in soliciting their life stories, thereby partly determining who writes an autobiography. Likewise, market issues can play an important role in determining the nature of the autobiographical account, for example, with public "confessions" or "kiss-and-tell" accounts promulgating the current market. Here, the introspective or social value of the autobiography may be confounded by the economic motive.

Note that the previous discussion applies only to publicly accessible *written* autobiographies. It does not tell us much about the true status of the *autobiographical process* throughout history.

Autobiography and the "Common Man"

It might be argued that in contrast to the public account of one's life, the autobiographical process itself (i.e., life review) is a nearly universal activity of humankind. Early in history, while the written word was reserved for the chosen few, the accounts of a family elder in spoken reminiscence was an essential part of culture. In the absence of a public educational system, people generally relied on their predecessors' stories for information necessary to survival and for transmitting the rules of acceptance into their social structure. Older adults in particular were valued for their rich experiential base.

Likewise, with little or no access to current forms of entertainment, storytelling was a popular practice. Many stories were likely to be based on personal recollections or transmitted family history. This retelling of the past was and is essential to the development and maintenance of family structure and constitutes a role most often filled by the older-adult grandparent (Knipscheer, 1988).

Life review employs reminiscence, a basic function of memory essential to mental well-being and human development. Individuals can interpret the world around them only in the context of the self, developing a cognitive organization or world view based more on personal interpretation than on objective events (Greenwald, 1980; Thomae, 1970; Wrightsman, 1980). Interpretation of events is in turn based on a review of past events as already interpreted by the self, that is, on reminiscence. Thus, the ego, or self, can be seen as the "organization of knowledge" (Greenwald, 1980). People engage in reminiscence on a daily basis and record current events as personal history. "Because reminiscing generally becomes 'second nature' after seven years of age, people lose sight of its subtle operation" (Magee, 1988, p. 1).

> Life review has the same immediate, fluid nature that characterizes reminiscence. It is a form of reminiscence in which individuals reflect upon their personal history and accept responsibility for it. It is a process in which reviewers gradually reconstruct and assess their past, using their current values to weigh behavior that their memories progressively return to consciousness. (Magee, 1988, p. 4)

From this perspective, one could argue that to some extent life review is an ongoing, universal process necessary to personal development and successful adaptation. Particularly in times of decision, a structured life review can play a vital role in assisting the person in analyzing choices and projecting future outcomes.

Older Adults' Interest in the Autobiography Process

Researchers and scholars in the field of adult development and aging generally agree that many older persons have an interest in life review. It thus appeared worthwhile to investigate the level of interest in autobiography by the older adults (Birren, Fisher, and Deutchman, 1988). A subject sample of college-educated older adults was chosen, representing over 6,000 alumni who graduated fifty or more years ago from the University of Southern California in Los Angeles.

A subsample of 3,095 of this group living in the Los Angeles and Orange counties was sent a questionnaire. There were 524 completed questionnaires returned. Approximately 50 additional were returned with a note indicating that the alumni was deceased or unable to complete the questionnaire.

Of the completed questionnaires that were returned, twenty-nine percent (29%) indicated an interest in autobiography. This number is impressive, since the request for information was the first time an initiative of a participatory character had been proposed to this subject sample.

In response to this survey, many alumni contacted the authors, demonstrating a strong desire to begin their autobiographies. This demonstrated high interest has led to the development of ongoing autobiography groups among university alumni. Reasons given for wanting to write an autobiographical account of one's history, despite no plans to publish it, fall into four primary categories: (1) to provide a legacy to be passed on to one's children, grandchildren, or both, (2) to review one's life achievements and prepare for the next steps, (3) to develop friendships, and (4) to engage in a creative process. A few participants also have expressed an interest in expanding the autobiographical statements written for the group into full-length autobiographies, with the potential of publishing their life stories. It is likely that university-educated older adults have a higher interest in autobiography than the less well educated. The correlates of autobiographical interest, however, are not known in detail and warrant study so we can serve better the aging population.

Table 9-1 describes the results of this survey. Note that most respondents were male, aged 70 to 79, and professionals. Of those interested in autobiography, men and women were found to be about equally interested. Although the best predictor of interest in autobiography was found to be interest in creative writing (70%), occupational differences were noted.

For the purpose of data analysis, occupation was coded into four categories: homemaker, technical, business, and professional. Engineers were coded as a technical occupation; educators, attorneys, physicians, dentists, and architects were coded as professionals; the business category included insurance brokers, certified public accountants, managers, and business owners; and homemakers were persons who did not specifically pursue a career. Professionals were found to be more likely to be interested in autobiography, whereas those who pursued a technical career were least likely to be interested (see Table 9-1).

Table 9-1. Age, Gender, and Occupation by Level
of Interest in Autobiography (percent)

	Percent Interested	Percent Not Interested
Age		
70–79	31	69
80–89	32	68
90+	39	61
Sex		
Male	40	60
Female	38	62
Occupation		
Homemaker	23	77
Technical	17	83
Business	28	72
Professional	37	63
College Major		
Business	33	67
Liberal Arts	33	67
Natural Sciences	26	74
Social Sciences	31	69
Education	41	59
Interest in Creative Writing	70	30

Reprinted with permission from Birren, Fisher, and
Deutchman, 1988.

The Uses of Autobiographical Accounts in Research

Autobiography as a tool for scientific research was early described by
Allport (1942). It has been used as a source of data and insights into human development (Borenstein, 1983; Lieberman and Falk, 1971) and the
human condition and social change (Roos, 1985; Wachter, 1988). The use
of autobiographies in the research process spans a number of disciplines,
including psychology, sociology, anthropology, history, literary criticism,
and political science. It is particularly relevant to cross-disciplinary research
which attempts to uncover the interaction between individual and environment or social structure (Bertaux and Kohli, 1984). The primary value
of using autobiographies in research is that they can provide an inner view
of the person not accessible through other methods of data collection.

The high degree of acceptance of autobiography as a data source in early behavioral and social research is most exemplified by research conducted in Poland just prior to the post–World War II Marxist era. During this period, two Polish sociologists developed a program of data collection whereby public competitions soliciting theme-related memoirs were held (Bertaux and Kohli, 1984). These competitions were announced in newspapers and resulted in the collection of thousands of autobiographical statements on select themes, for example, the life of a peasant. The best were published in books. These memoirs provided a rich source of data for sociological research and were used by many Polish investigators.

As Bertaux and Kohli (1984) indicated, however, scholarly interest in these data in the behavioral sciences waned somewhat over the last two decades, reemerging only recently. The reasons for this decline and the subsequent reemergence of personal documents as a source of data are discussed below.

The Emergence of Behaviorism

Key to the decline in the use of personal documents as a data source in scientific research was the rise of behaviorism and its methodological reservations regarding their subjective nature. Central to their subsequent reemergence were increased acknowledgment of the importance of subjectivity in understanding the organization of behavior in the person and realization of the vital role personal statements can play in research designed to explore the interaction between events, individual interpretation, and behavior. A similar trajectory was followed in the social sciences (particularly anthropology and sociology), with the use of personal documents peaking in the heyday of the Chicago School, declining during the era dominated by the survey method, and reemerging only recently (Roos, 1988).

In the heyday of behaviorism, its exclusive focus on "observables" as the only methodologically sound form of data left little room for the analysis of retrospective accounts, life review, or reminiscence. The reality of subjectivity itself as a major factor in human development was ignored, and increased understanding of human behavior was limited to overt behavior that could be counted and quantified.

As a proponent of behaviorism, Holt (1962) questioned the representativeness of personal data and suggested that useful information was impossible to gain, since the transfer of findings from one case to another was limited. Nunnally (1978) posited that the use of these data would represent an antiscience point of view in that its use discouraged the search for general laws and instead favored the description of particular phenomena.

Questions concerning the reliability of these data were studied in longitudinal research comparing a person's account of an event at the time of its occurrence and his or her account some time after. For example, Kent (1985) found that dental patients' reports of acute pain obtained three months after a procedure were significantly different from those same patients' reports immediately following the procedure. Specifically, patients characterized as anxious reported more pain at follow-up than they had previously reported.

What the proponents of behaviorism missed, however, is that such distortion is itself a feature of behavior. It confounds research only to the extent that the goal of investigation is solely an objective account of a past event. "Social and behavioral scientists typically are not historians in this sense. That is, the aim is not to recreate the past, but rather to understand the past from the perspective of the present" (de Vries, Deutchman, and Birren, in press).

This point is particularly relevant in the case of behavioral research that seeks to uncover factors that influence human development and behavior. For example, in Kent's study of dental patients, one might argue that the findings not only shed light on the reliability of personal accounts but also demonstrated the effects of anxiety on perception and, possibly, the impact of this anxiety on future behaviors, for example, utilization of dental health services. In this context, individual interpretation and the biases that accompany it may instead be seen as representative of cognitive organization (Greenwald, 1980), or world views, which could arguably have more impact on human development and personality than the actual objective events (Wrightsman, 1980), as is seen in William's example:

> William joined the guided autobiography sessions in the hope of understanding and mastering a life-long apprehension about public speaking. His anxiety was based in a belief that he was unable to present himself well verbally and should maintain a career position that relied primarily on written reports. It prevented William from accepting a promotion to a managerial position that would greatly increase the economic security of his family. The managerial position would require monthly presentations by William to a group of investors.
>
> In reviewing his life story, William recounted his family his-

tory as the youngest of five children. He recalled a number of incidents from his childhood that centered around his parents' approval of him as the "quiet, studious one" and of his brother as "outgoing." As a child, he interpreted this as a sign that his parents had little confidence in his verbal communication style and viewed him as less popular. The guided autobiography group leader, with the assistance of other members, encouraged William to reassess these events as an adult. In doing so, William recognized that they were relatively minor comments, and he developed a new perspective that focused on his parents' desire to develop a sense of individuality among their children. He recognized that the interpretation he placed on minor events of his childhood had a negative and unnecessary impact on his self-esteem and decision making.

William's story highlights the important role of personal interpretation of events and relationships as a primary factor in both behavioral and emotional development. It demonstrates that a person's emotional or affective weighing of events may change over time, influencing interpretation and future action; it emphasizes the importance of affect in understanding human development. In the study of the organization of behavior, personal accounts represent an important and reliable data source in research designed to study affect and its interaction with cognition and behavior. To the issues of personal interpretation and affect might be added beliefs, which have a strong impact on behavior. An example of research designed to utilize autobiographies in this way is that by Cornwell and Geering (1989), which seeks to understand health beliefs and the impact of these beliefs on the health behaviors of older adults and their response to illness.

In support of using personal documents in research, Thomae (1970, p. 70) developed two postulates of human behavior: (1) "perception of change rather than objective change is related to behavioral change" and (2) "any change in the situation of the individual is perceived and evaluated in terms of the dominant concerns and expectations of the individual." This perhaps represents the underlying reasoning of Freud who developed many of his psychological theories by listening to his patient's personal accounts of their lives (de Vries, Deutchman and Birren, in press). Likewise, Hall (1922) and Murray (1938) used diaries and autobiographies in the development of their seminal theories of adult development and personality, respectively.

Methodological Issues

Criticisms of the use of autobiographical data in research generally address one of three methodological concerns: (1) reliability and representativeness of the data; (2) what Gaston (1982) termed "problems of conceptualization of the data," focusing on experimenter biases and flexibility and reliability of data analysis; and (3) accuracy of reporting. Although these concerns are valid and must be taken into account in research design, methods exist to address these issues, and the value of this research should not be overlooked.

Reliability and Representativeness

The first concern was earlier expressed in the views of Nunnally, who saw the study of the individual or the idiographic approach as an antiscience. He based his argument on the proposition that this approach necessarily "discourages the search for general laws and instead encourages description of particular phenomena (people)" (Nunnally, 1978, p. 548). This criticism, however, defies scientific precedent, ignoring the usefulness of analyzing the organism at the level of the individual's experience. This analysis holds rich potential for explorations not only into understanding individual behavior but also into issues of interindividual development and change.

Runyan (1984), a strong proponent of the study of psychology and autobiography, drew a parallel between behavioral research that focuses on the individual and similar research in other domains, for example, geological research focusing on the structure and evolution of the earth, excluding other planets. He posited that quantitative and experimental studies of the single case hold great potential for understanding human development at the level of the individual. Similarities and differences can then be drawn between cases in the service of theory construction to address general factors that influence personal development.

Problems of Conceptualization

According to Gaston (1982), problems of a priori conceptualization may have an impact on the reliability and, thereby, the usefulness of autobiographical data in two ways: (1) Investigators' preconceived hypotheses may influence their interpretation of the data in such a way that they ignore aspects of the data that do not directly relate to their a priori position.

In this way, alternative explanations of the data are missed, and interpretation is subjugated to the investigator's already existing conceptual framework. (2) Studies using idiographic data may be irrelevant due to poorly formulated or ambiguous methodologies. This approach raises questions of inter-rater reliability, may leave the data open to misinterpretation due to investigator biases, and potentially renders the research unavailable for replication. Careful design of research, however, can bypass such problems, generating meaningful results that would otherwise be unobtainable.

Gaston (1982) noted two methods of data analysis that avoid problems of conceptualization. The first method, analytic induction, has been described by Denzin (1970). In this method, the researcher begins with a hypothesis that serves as an explanation of the phenomenon in question. After examining the first case, a decision is made as to whether or not the hypothesis holds true for that case. If the hypothesis does not hold true, it is reformulated so that the information gained from the case is explained. This new hypothesis is then tested against the next case, and so on. As the analysis progresses, each case is evaluated in regard to the immediate hypothesis generated by testing the previous case. The goal of this methodology is to generate a universal explanation of all data in the sample.

The second methodology suggested by Gaston is the constant comparative method developed by Glaser and Strauss (1967). In this method, the hypothesis is derived initially from the body of data itself rather than from a preconceived hypothesis taken by the experimenter approaching the data. This is accomplished through the development of categories, the basic unit of analysis in the constant comparative method. Categories are constructed from the data by fitting each piece of information in the data into as many categories as possible. Categories become better defined and more distinct as the analysis progresses. Hypotheses are then generated by describing the relationships that emerge among the categories. The theory is then constructed to explain the interconnections among the hypotheses.

A criticism of these two methods is that "conclusions are only universal to the extent that cases that invalidate them are not yet identified" (Birren and Hedlund, 1987). This problem can be overcome through subsequent investigation and replication.

Accuracy of Reporting

Of special concern in the use of autobiographical data is the degree to which people are accurate reporters of their lives. This is true of any self-report measure in that the possibility exists for subjects, consciously or unconsciously, to withhold or color the information they provide. Research designed to assess the scope of this problem, however, indicates that such data are generally valid. Subjects do not tend to intentionally color their reports. Information that diverges from reality generally represents valid and reliable insight into the world view of the individual.

Shaffer (1954) examined the accuracy of five hundred autobiographical statements and found that deception was used in only 3% of the documents, in terms of gross exaggerations, internal inconsistencies, or improbabilities of life events. Regarding the honesty of "objective" data, for example, data of birth, which could be verified through other records, 99% of the autobiographical statements were found to be accurate.

Lieberman and Falk (1971), in a study utilizing 180 aged and 25 middle-aged persons, sought to determine if reminiscence data would provide a source of pertinent constructs for understanding adult development. They concluded that reminiscence is an important source of data for developing a psychology of the life span, and they called for further research and theory development in this vital area.

The Current Uses and Potential for Future Research

Recent articles in professional journals, the well-stocked shelves of bookstores, and the increased attention of the media attest to the reemergence of autobiography as a major source of contemporary literature and a focal point for understanding human development. Autobiography's reemergence is particularly evident in the increase of literature on the subject in such journals as the *Chronicle of Higher Education* and *Biography*, an interdisciplinary quarterly. Birren and Hedlund (1987) posit that this reemergence is a reflection of the *zeitgeist* of a changing society in which the brain is regarded as a complex organism encompassing cognition, connation, and affect, rather than simply malleable material organized into piles of data as a function of environmental contingencies. Both the "hardware" and the "software" of the nervous system are taken seriously, as are the statements that people make about their development. Autobiographical materials are now recognized as important to understanding the processes of growing up and growing old, providing clues that might not otherwise be readily available solely by observations of overt behavior.

The value of autobiographical data for research is not limited to studies that focus on individual development. The reemergence of the use of such data also has been noted in the social sciences and the humanities. For example, as will be discussed below, personal statements can represent an irreplaceable source of data for understanding social history in light of its impact on people.

Behavioral Sciences

To understand fully the current use of autobiographical data in the behavioral sciences, it is important to trace its roots in theory development. Many of the seminal theories that still shape scientific thought were, at least in part, derived from analyzing personal statements. For example, G. S. Hall, one of the founders of child psychology early in the twentieth century, used diaries and autobiographies as a source of data in the construction of his theories on adolescence (as cited in Annis, 1967). Freud developed many of his psychological constructs by listening to the lives, accounts, and experiences of his patients (de Vries, Deutchman, Birren, in press). And Murray (1938) used diaries and autobiographies along with twenty-eight other assessment techniques in constructing his theories of personality. Table 9-2 notes just some of the behavioral scientists who have used autobiographical data in the service of theory development to dem-

Table 9-2. Behavioral Scientists Who Have Used Autobiographical Data in the Service of Theory Development

Research Scientist	Theory
Birren and Hedlund (1987)	The development of meaning
Buhler and Massarik (1968)	The development of values
Frenkel (1936)	Life-span development
Freedman (1974)	Cognitive disturbances in schizophrenia
Hall (1922)	Adolescence
Levinson, Darrow, Klein, Levinson, and McKee (1978)	Adult development
Lowenthal, Thurnher, and Chiriboga (1975)	The development of coping strategies
Murray (1938)	Personality
White (1952)	Personality

onstrate its widespread influence on the history and future of behavioral research.

Murray (1938, p. 39) may have put it best when he argued that "the history of the organism is the organism." Table 9-2 lists just some of the behavioral theorists who agree with this view of human behavior and rely on autobiographical data to access this important aspect of the individual. Perhaps we should add to Murray's statement the thought that the individual's interpretation of history, as well as history itself, is the individual.

Another area that relies on autobiographical data for much of its research is counseling psychology. In fact, Birren and Hedlund (1987) pointed out that this area has shown the largest increase in the last decades of studies utilizing autobiographical data. Examples of such research include studies of adjustment (Shaffer, 1954) and assessment of vocational and personal needs (Cottle and Downie, 1960; Hahn and MacLean, 1955; Riccio, 1958; Tyler, 1953).

In addition, research directed at clinical treatment has proposed autobiographical data as a means of increasing insight on the part of counselors (Baird, 1957; Tolbert, 1959) and of providing meaningful services to older adults (Bratter and Tuvman, 1980; Butler and Lewis, 1982). An example of these services was presented by Greene (1982) in her analysis of life review as a technique for clarifying family roles in adulthood. Greene found that in addition to providing a sense of meaning of life as it has been lived, life review can assist the older adult in adjustment to retirement, shifts in parental responsibility, and renegotiation of relationships with family and spouse. A more complete discussion of the potential therapeutic outcomes of life review was presented above in Chapter 1. Of importance here is that the autobiographical process itself has become not only a way to research adult development but also a way to influence adjustment and meaning over the life cycle.

Social Sciences

Use of autobiographical data in the social sciences spans almost every area and is particularly relevant to sociology, anthropology, and political science.

Sociology

Bertaux and Kohli (1984) pointed to the importance of autobiographical statements and oral life stories as a way of addressing the substantive, or theoretical, questions of sociology. They noted that many contemporary sociologists use these data to investigate some set of social relationships (e.g., Bertaux and Bertaux-Wiame, 1981; Carmargo, 1981; Kohli, 1982; Thompson, 1983) and that the same could be said for most anthropological studies. They reasoned that this interest is due to the efforts taken by most social sciences to understand sociohistorical processes in which both action and subjectivity play a part.

Bertaux and Kohli (1984) noted two areas of sociological research in which life stories play a particularly important role: (1) the cultural or life-world approach to Marxism, for example, research on class consciousness (Alheit, 1983; Bahrdt, 1975; Brose, 1983; Osterland, 1978) and (2) phenomenological or interpretive research on the life course and socialization (Kohli, 1978; Rosenmayr, 1981). Of particular relevance is the importance of autobiographical data in research aimed at understanding the impact of social history on personal development (e.g., Kohli, Rosenow, and Wolf, 1983), as well as the "sociocultural changes that take place in the development of individuality" (Roos, 1988, p. 3).

> Bill grew up in a small American town in the years just follow-
> ing World War II. In participating in the guided autobiography
> group, Bill recounted the difficulties of being a Japanese-American
> during those years. He remarked on the stress young boys, like
> himself, put on proving they were, indeed, American. During
> his youth, Bill rejected many of his family's traditions and fo-
> cused his energies on all he perceived as appropriate to the "typi-
> cal American teenager." Many of his life-long skills and interests,
> for example in sports and technology, were an outgrowth of
> those developmental years, which were indelibly marked by the
> social climate.

Ethnomethodology is a third area of sociological research in which autobiographical data plays a vital role. According to Benson and Hughes (1983, p. 30), ethnomethodology is research aimed at "the ordinary, common-sense, mundane world in which members live and do so in a way that remains faithful to the methods, procedures, practices, etc., that members themselves use in constructing and making sense of this social world." This area of research thereby seeks data that illuminate individuals' perceptions and experiences of the world around them; the perceptions and interpretations of everyday events and circumstances are the key sources of data, unlike other areas of science, which focus on objective events or the analysis of general principles across societies.

Anthropology

For the most part, anthropological research that draws on autobiography as a data source is rooted in the *life-history method*. This method involves obtaining life histories that are comprised of oral life stories supplemented with biographical data drawn from other sources, for example, court, medical, or psychological records (Bertaux, 1981). "The life-history method results in a view of the person's life that is a product of the interaction between the anthropologist and the individual in historical context" (Birren and Hedlund, 1987). One example of relevance to gerontological research is Myerhoff's (1978) book about an older-adult Jewish community in California, *Number Our Days*, which is the result of research utilizing the life-history method.

Political Science

In recent years, there has been a return to the use of autobiographical data from earlier periods to better understand political history and the role of the individual in the formation of public policy. Wachter's (1988) bibliography of works about life-writing contains many examples of how autobiographical statements can shed light on the political climate of bygone eras. Of particular importance is autobiographical data of women (e.g., Blanco, 1986; Geiger, 1986) and minority groups (e.g., Kim, 1987) who may have held little overt political power and may be otherwise disregarded in the political writings of their historical eras. Through the analysis of autobiographical statements, one can gain a new perspective on both the ofttimes covert roles these groups played in the formation of policy and social change and the impact of policies on persons.

An example of the use of autobiographical data in research of this kind is Alonso and Baranda's (1980) study of refugees from the Spanish Civil War, which seeks to understand political exile and its consequences. Likewise, a large-scale project at the Centro de Pesquisa e Documentaçao of the Fundaçao Getulio Varga in Rio de Janeiro traces the histories of the Brazilian elites from the 1930s to 1964 and has been used to analyze the processes of elite recruitment, internal division of elites, and policymaking (Carmargo, 1981, as cited in Bertaux and Kohli, 1984).

Humanities

The humanities traditionally have been the most accepting of autobiography as a data source, being focused on the "totality of human beings"

(*Webster's Third International Dictionary,* 1981). Its use spans the study of history, literature, theology, and the arts.

Autobiography provides a rich resource for understanding the impact of historical events on persons (e.g., see articles listed in Wachter, 1988). For example, Cole and Premo (1984) promoted the value of qualitative analyses of autobiographies written by persons over the age of 55 during the last 150 years; the purpose of this research is to understand the historical identities of older adults and to contrast these with the identities of older adults in today's society.

Autobiography also has been employed in the search for understanding the motivations and influences that form the perspective of the artist. For example, Rich (1988) demonstrated how the creative processes of writing and revising a novel can reflect key aspects of an author's life history. Similarly, Stout (1987) traced one author's use of biography as a creative medium that was part of a search for self-presence; the search, in turn, was an integral part of the artist's work.

It has been further posited that autobiography provides unique insight into issues of spiritual development and the role of religion in adaptation and maturation. For example, Hedlund (as cited in Birren and Hedlund, 1987) analyzed 145 autobiographical essays on the topic of meaning in life and found that the item "religious or individual belief system" was among the four major categories of life meaning (i.e., altruism or service, personal growth, personal relationships, and beliefs).

Thus, the literature supports the view that autobiography provides unique insight into the internal world of the individual. Guided autobiography is an irreplaceable resource for understanding that world, preparing the individual for the future.

References

Alheit, P. 1983. *Alltagsleben: Zur Bedentung eines gesellschaftlichen "Restphanomens."* Frankfort: Campus.

Allport, G. 1942. *The use of personal documents in psychological science* (Bull. 49). Social Science Research Council.

Alonso, M. S., and Baranda, M. 1980. *Palabros del exilio.* Mexico City: Institute of National Anthropology.

Alpaugh, P., and Birren, J. E. 1977. Variables affecting creative contributions across the life span. *Human Development* 20: 240–48.

Anderson, R. 1970. *I never sang for my father.* New York: New American Library.

Annis, A. P. 1967. The autobiography: Its uses and value in professional psychology. *Journal of Counseling Psychology* 14 (1): 9–17.

Bahrdt, H. P. 1975. Erzahlte Lebensgeschichten von Arbeitern. In M. Osterland, ed., *Arbeitsituation, Lebensbilanzen, und Lebensperspektiven von Industriearbeitern.* Frankfort: Europaische Verlagsanstalt.

Baird, C. R. 1957. The autobiography. *Education Digest* 19: 39–43.

Benson, D., and Hughes, J. A. 1983. *The perspective of ethnomethodology.* New York: Longman.

Berg, S., and Ruth, J. E. 1982. Creativity in old age: A longitudinal study. *Aging, Clinical and Experimental Research,* 2–13.

Berghorn, F. J., and Schafer, D. E. 1987. Reminiscence intervention in nursing homes: What and who changes? *International Journal of Aging and Human Development* 24 (2): 113–27.

Bertaux, D. 1981. *Biography and society.* Berkeley, Calif.: Sage Publications.

Bertaux, D., and Bertaux-Wiame, I. 1981. Life stories in the baker's trade. In D. Bertaux, ed., *Biography and society.* Berkeley, Calif.: Sage Publications.

Bertaux, D., and Kohli, M. 1984. The life story approach: A continental view. *Annual Review of Sociology* 10: 215–37.

Birren, J. E. 1990. Creativity, productivity, and potentials of the senior scholar. *Gerontology and Geriatrics Education.* Forthcoming.

Birren, J. E. In press. Spiritual maturity in psychological development. *Journal of Religion and Aging.*

Birren, J. E., Fisher, L. M., and Deutchman, D. E. 1988. "Older adult interest in personal history and autobiography: A survey of elderly college educated adults." Unpublished manuscript. University of Southern California.

Birren, J. E., and Hedlund, B. 1987. Contributions of autobiography to developmental psychology. In N. Eisenberg, ed., *Contemporary topics in developmental psychology*, 394–415. New York: John Wiley.

Birren, J. E., Hoppe, C., and Birren, B. "Identity and autobiography." Unpublished manuscript. University of Southern California.

Blanco, A. 1986. In their chosen place: On the autobiographies of two Spanish women of the left. *Genre* 19: 431–45.

Borenstein, A. 1983. *Chimes of change and hours.* London: Associated University Press.

Botwinick, J. 1978. *Aging and behavior.* 2nd ed. New York: Springer.

Boylin, W., Gordon, S. K., and Nehrke, M. F. 1976. Reminiscing and ego integrity in institutionalized elderly males. *Gerontologist* 16: 118–24.

Bratter, T. E., and Tuvman, E. 1980. A peer counseling program in action. In S. Stansfeld Sargent, ed., *Nontraditional therapy and counseling with the aged.* New York: Springer.

Brose, H. G. 1983. *Die Erfahrung der Arbeit: Zum berufsbiographischen Eraverb von Handlungsmustern bei Industriearbeitern.* Opladen, West Germany: Verlag.

Buhler, C., Massarik, F. 1968. *The course of human life.* New York: Springer.

Bumagin, V. E., and Hirn, K. F. 1990. *Helping the aging family: A guide for professionals.* Glenview, Ill.: Scott, Foresman.

Burnside, I. 1984. *Working with the elderly: Group processes and techniques.* Belmont, Calif.: Wadsworth.

Burnside, I. 1988. *Nursing and the aged: A self-care approach.* 3rd ed. New York: McGraw-Hill.

Butler, R. N. 1963. The life review: An interpretation of reminiscence in old age. *Psychiatry, Journal for the Study of Inter-Personal Processes* 26: 65–76.

Butler, R. N. 1967. Studies of creative people and the creative process after middle life. In S. Levin and R. H. Kahana, eds., *Psychodynamic studies on aging.* New York: International University Press.

Butler, R. N., and Lewis, M. I. 1982. *Aging and mental health,* 3rd ed., St. Louis: Mosby.

Carmargo, A. 1981. The actor and the system: Trajectory of Brazilian elites. In D. Bertaux, ed., *Biography and Society.* Berkeley, Calif.: Sage Publications.

Cole, T. R., and Premo, T. 1984. "Aging in American autobiography: Meaning, identity and history." Unpublished manuscript. University of Texas.

Coleman, P. G. 1974. "The role of the past in adaptation to old age." Ph.D. diss., University of London.

Coleman, P. G. 1986. *Aging and reminiscence processes: Social and clinical implications.* New York: John Wiley.

Cornwell, J., and Geering, B. 1989. Biographical interviews with older people. *Oral History Journal* 1: 36–43.

Costa, P. T., and Kastenbaum, R. 1967. Some aspects of memories and ambitions in centenarians. *Journal of Genetic Psychology* 100: 3–16.

Cottle, W. C., and Downie, N. M. 1960. *Procedures and preparation for counseling.* Englewood Cliffs, N.J.: Prentice-Hall.

Denzin, N. K. 1970. *The research act.* Chicago: Aldine.

de Vries, B., Deutchman, D. E., and Birren, J. E. 1990. Adult development through guided autobiography: The family context. *Family Educations Journal* 39: 3–7.

Ebersole, P. P. 1978. Establishing reminiscing groups. In I. M. Burnside, ed., *Working with the elderly: Group processes and techniques.* North Sciutate, Mass.: Duxbury.

Elbaz, R. 1988. *The changing nature of the self: A critical study of the autobiographic discourse.* London: Croom Helm.

Erickson, E. H. 1963. *Childhood and society,* 2nd ed. New York: Norton.

Freedman, B. 1974. The subjective experience of perceptual and cognitive disturbances in schizophrenia. *Archives of General Psychiatry* 30: 333–40.

Frenkel, E. 1936. Studies in biographical psychology. *Character & Personality* 5: 1–34.

Gaston, C. 1982. The use of personal documents in the study of adulthood. Paper presented at the annual meeting of the American Psychological Association, Washington, D.C., August.

Geiger, S. N. 1986. Women's life histories: Method and content. *Signs,* Winter, 334–51.

Georgemiller, R., and Maloney, H. N. 1984. Group life review and denial of death. *Clinical Gerontologist* 2 (4): 37–49.

Glaser, B., and Strauss, A. 1967. *The discovery of grounded theory: Strategies for qualitative research.* Chicago: Aldine.

Goldwasser, A., Auerbach, S. M., and Harkins, S. W. 1987. Cognitive, affective, and behavioral effects of reminiscence group therapy on demented elderly. *International Journal of Aging and Human Development* 25 (3): 209–22.

Gould, Roger L. 1978. *Transformations: Growth and change in adult life.* New York: Simon & Schuster.

Greene, R. R. 1982. Life review: A technique for clarifying family roles in adulthood. *Clinical Gerontologist* 1 (2): 59–67.

Greenwald, A. 1980. The totalitarian ego: Fabrication and revision of personal history. *American Psychologist* 35: 603–18.

Grotjahn, M. L. 1989. Group analysis in old age. *Group Analysis* 22: 109–11.

Hahn, M. E., and MacLean, M. S. 1955. *Counseling psychology.* New York: McGraw-Hill.

Hall, G. S. 1922. *Senescence, the last half of life.* New York: Appleton, Century, Crofts.

Hately, B. J. 1985. Spiritual well-being through life histories. *Journal of Religion & Aging* 1 (2): 63–71.

Havighurst, R. J., and Glaser, R. 1972. An exploratory study of reminiscence. *Journal of Gerontology* 27: 245–53.

Holt, R. R. 1962. Individuality and generalization in the psychology of personality. *Journal of Personality* 30: 377–404.

Hughston, G., and Merriam, S. 1982. Reminiscence: A nonformal technique for improving cognitive functioning in the aged. *Journal of Aging and Human Development* 15: 139–49.

Ingersoll, B., and Silverman, A. 1978. Comparative group psychotherapy for the aged. *Gerontologist* 18: 201–6.

Kaminsky, M. 1978. Pictures from the past: The use of reminiscence in casework with the elderly. *Journal of Gerontological Social Work* 1 (1): 19–29.

Kent, G. 1985. Memory of dental pain. *Pain* 21: 187–94.

Kim, S. G. 1987. Black Americans' commitment to communism: A case study based on fiction and autobiographies by Black Americans. *Dissertation Abstracts,* 48: 3415–6B. University of Kansas.

Knipscheer, C. P. M. 1988. Temporal embeddedness and aging within the multi-generational family: The case of grandparenting. In J. E. Birren and V. L. Bengtson, eds., *Emergent theories of aging.* New York: Springer.

Kohli, M. 1978. *Soziologie des Lebenslaufs.* Darmstadt, West Germany: Luchterhand.

Kohli, M. 1982. "Biographical research in German language area. Ad hoc group on the 'Uses of autobiographical narratives,'" 10th World Congress of Sociology, Mexico, 16–21 August.

Kohli, M., Rosenow, J., and Wolf, J. 1983. The social construction of aging through work: Economic structure and life-world. *Aging and Society* 3: 23–42.

Leedy, J. 1969. *Poetry therapy: Use of poetry in the treatment of emotional disorders.* Philadelphia: J. B. Lippincott.

Lejeune, P. 1986. *Moi aussi.* Paris: Editions du Seuil (as cited in Roos, 1986).

Levinson, D. J., Darrow, C. N., Klein, E. B., Levinson, M. H., and McKee, B. 1978. *The seasons of a man's life.* New York: Knopf.

Lewis, M. I. 1973. The adaptive value of reminiscing in old age. *Journal of Geriatric Psychiatry* 6: 117–21.

Lewis, M. I., and Butler, R. 1974. Life-review therapy: Putting memories to work in individual and group psychotherapy. *Geriatrics* November: 165–69.

Lieberman, M. A., and Falk, J. M. 1971. The remembered past as a source of data for research on the life cycle. *Human Development* 14: 132–41.

Lowenthal, M., Thurnher, M., and Chiriboga, D. 1975. *Four Stages of Life.* San Francisco: Jossey-Bass.

Maddi, S. R. 1970. The search for meaning. *Proceedings of the Nebraska Symposium on Motivation.* Lincoln: University of Nebraska Press.

Magee, J. J. 1988. *A professional's guide to older adults' life review.* Lexington, Mass.: Lexington Books.

McMahon, A. W., and Rhudick, P. J. 1967. Reminiscing in the aged: An adaptational response. In S. Levin and R. J. Kahana, eds. *Psychodynamic studies on aging: Creativity, reminiscing and dying.* New York: International University Press.

Murray, H. A. 1938. *Explorations in personality.* New York: Oxford University Press.

Myerhoff, B. G. 1978. *Number our days.* New York: Touchstone.

Myerhoff, B. G., and Tufte, V. 1975. Life history as integration: Personal myth and aging. *Gerontologist* 15: 541–43.

Nunnally, J. C. 1978. *Psychometric theory*. 2nd ed. New York: McGraw-Hill.

Olney, J. 1980. *Autobiography: Essays theoretical and critical*. Princeton, N.J.: Princeton University Press.

Osterland, M. 1978. *Lebensperspektiven von Industriearbeitern*. Neuwied, West Germany: Luchterhand.

Price, C. 1983. Heritage: A program design for reminiscence. *Activities, Adaptation & Aging* 3 (3): 47–53.

Progoff, I. 1975. *At a journal workshop*. New York: Dialogue House Library.

Reedy, M. N., and Birren, J. E. 1980. *Life review through autobiography*. Poster session presented at annual meeting of American Psychological Association, Montreal.

Riccio, A. C. 1958. The status of the autobiography. *Peabody Journal of Education* 36: 33–36.

Rich, S. L. 1988. Mirror, mirror: An autobiographical study in creative process. *Dissertation Abstracts* 48: 1766A. New York University.

Roos, J. P. 1985. Life stories of social changes: Four generations in Finland. *International Journal of Oral History* 6 (3): 179–90.

Roos, J. P. 1988. *Elamantavasta elamakertaan*, Gymmerus, OY: Zyvaskyla (139–54).

Rosenmayr, L. 1981. Objective and subjective perspectives of life span research. *Aging and Society* 1: 29–49.

Runyan, W. M. 1984. *Life histories and psychobiography: Exploratories in theory and method*. New York: Oxford University Press.

Ruth, J. E., and Birren, J. E. 1985. Creativity in adulthood and old age: Relations to intelligence, sex and mode of testing. *International Journal of Behavioral Dvelopment* 8: 99–109.

Sarbin, T. R. 1986. *Narrative psychology: The storied nature of human conduct*. New York: Praeger.

Selling, B. 1989. *Writing from within*. Claremont, Calif.: Hunter House.

Shaffer, E. E. 1954. The autobiography in secondary counseling. *Personnel & Guidance Journal* 32: 395–98.

Shute, G. E. 1986. Life review: A cautionary note. *Clinical Gerontologist* 6 (1): 57–58.

Sperbeck, D. J., Whitbourne, S. K., and Hoyer, W. J. 1986. Age and openness to experience in autobiographical memory. *Experimental Aging Research* 12 (3): 169–72.

Stout, J. C. 1987. Antonin Artaud as a writer of biographies. *Dissertation Abstracts* 48: 936A. Princeton University.

Summers, H. 1970. High school photograph with calendar, courtesy of Lamborn's, Athens, Ohio. *Sit opposite each other*. New Jersey: Rutgers University Press. Copyright © 1970 by Rutgers, The State University of New Jersey.

Thomae, H. 1970. Theory of aging and cognitive theory of personality. *Human Development* 13: 1–16.

Thompson, P. 1983. *Living the fishing*. London: Routledge & Kegan Paul.

Tolbert, E. L. 1959. *Introduction to counseling*. New York: McGraw-Hill.

Tyler, L. E. 1953. *The work of the counselor*. New York: Appleton, Century, Crofts.

Vaillant, G. 1971. *Adaptation to life*. Boston: Little, Brown.

Wachter, P. E. 1988. Current bibliography of life-writing. *Biography: An Interdisciplinary Quarterly* 11 (4): 316–25.

Webster's New International Dictionary. 2nd ed. 1971. Springfield, Mass.: G & C. Webster.

Webster's Third New International Dictionary. 1981. Springfield, Mass.: G & C. Webster.

Weintraub, K. J. 1978. *The value of the individual*. Chicago: University of Chicago Press.

White, R. R. 1952. *Lives in progress*. New York: Holt, Rinehart, & Winston.

Willis, S. L., and Schaie, K. W. 1985. "Ability correlates of real life tasks in young and later adulthood." Paper presented at the meetings of the Gerontological Society of America, New Orleans.

Wrightsman, L. S. 1980. "Personal documents as data in conceptualizing adult personality development." Presidential address to the Society of Personality and Social Psychology, American Psychological Association, Montreal.

Wrightsman, L. S. 1988. *Personality development in adulthood*. Beverly Hills, Calif.: Sage Publishers.

Yalom, I. D. 1975. *Existential psychotherapy*. New York: Basic Books.

Index

Absenteeism, 35, 39
Acceptance, mutual: in guided autobiography groups, 36–37, 48–49
Adaptation: to change, 20–22; cohort interaction and, 55–56; continuity and, 15–16; guided autobiography and, 1, 5
Adjustment. *See* Mental health
Adult education: guided autobiography as tool in, 6
Affect. *See* Emotions
Age: autobiographical writing and, 116; cautiousness and, 82; creativity and, 81–82; vocabulary and, 81–82
Agitation: depression and, 99
Alheit, P., 129, 133
Allport, G., 5, 116, 120, 133
Alonso, M. S., 130, 133
Alpaugh, P., 133
Altruism: as curative factor, 44–45
Amateur therapist, 97
Analytic induction, 125
Anderson, R., 22, 133
Annis, A. P., 5, 127, 133
Anonymity: in guided autobiography, 52–53
Anthropology: use of autobiographical data in, 120, 130
Anxiety: guided autobiography and, 14
Art: as theme of autobiographical writing, 77–78
Aspirations: as theme of autobiographical writing, 76–77
Audio taping: guided autobiography and, 84

Auerbach, S. M., 5, 135
Autobiography: "common man" and, 117–18; as a data source, 120–31; definition of, 108–9; history of, 114–18; motivation to write, 116–17; research on, 114–31; who writes, 114–20. *See also* Guided autobiography

Bahrdt, H. P., 129, 133
Baird, C. R., 128, 133
Baranda, M., 130, 133
Behavioral research: personal data and, 121–23, 127–28
Behaviorism: personal data and, 121–23
Belief system: identification of, through guided autobiography, 14–15
Benson, D., 129, 133
Bereavement, 48. *See also* Loss; Widowhood
Berg, S., 133
Berghorn, F. J., 5, 133
Bertaux, D., 120–21, 128–29, 130, 133–34
Bertaux-Wiame, I., 129, 133
Biography, 108–9, 126
Birren, B., 9, 134
Birren, J. E., 5, 9, 13–14, 81, 116, 118, 122, 123, 125, 126, 127, 128, 130, 131, 133, 134, 135, 137
Blanco, A., 130, 134
Body image: as theme of autobiographical writing, 72
Borenstein, A., 120, 134

Botwinick, J., 134
Boylin, W., 5, 14, 134
Branching points in life: as theme of autobiographical writing, 67–69
Bratter, T. E., 128, 134
Brose, H. G., 129
Buhler, C., 5, 12, 103–4, 127, 134
Bumagin, V. E., 99, 134
Burnside, I. M., 34, 134, 135
Butler, R. N., 1, 2, 5, 103, 128, 134, 136

Career: as theme of autobiographical writing, 70–71
Career group member, 96
Carmargo, A., 129, 130, 134
Catharsis: as curative factor, 44–45
Cautiousness: age and, 82
Change. See Outcomes of guided autobiography; Transitions
Chicago School, 121
Chiriboga, D., 127, 136
Choices: guided autobiography and, 7–9
Clark, T., 116, 134
Cognitive functioning: in group members, 34; guided autobiography and, 5, 19
Cohesiveness: as curative factor, 44–45; guided autobiography and, 62–63
Cohorts: in guided autobiography groups, 32–33; need for interaction within, 55–56
Cole, T. R., 130, 131, 134
Co-leaders, 28–29. See also Group leader
Coleman, P. G., 5, 98, 134
Competence. See Cognitive functioning; Self-efficacy
Confessions (St. Augustine), 115
Confidant: group leader as, 28; guided autobiography and, 55, 62–63; therapeutic role of, 3
Confidentiality: in guided autobiography process, 28, 52–53
Conflict. See Reconciliation
Confusion: depression and, 100
Constant comparative method, 125
Continuity in a life: guided autobiography and, 5, 14–17
Control: purpose fitness and, vii
Convergent thinking: definition of, 81

Coping: guided autobiography and, 5. See also Adaptation
Cornwell, J., 123, 134
Costa, P. T., 5, 14, 134
Costs of guided autobiography, 42–43
Cottle, W. C., 128, 135
Counseling: guided autobiography as tool in, 6
Creative writing, 108
Creativity: in guided autobiography, 80–93; metaphor and, 86–88; poetry and, 88–90; signs of, 80
Culture: mental health and, 15–17

Darrow, C. N., 127, 136
Death: guided autobiography and, 5, 22; life review and, 2; as theme of autobiographical writing, 74–75
Decision strategies: guided autobiography and, 6–9
Dementia: guided autobiography and, 34
Denzin, N. K., 125, 135
Depression: guided autobiography and, 5, 14; life review and, 99; planfulness and, 19; signs of, 98–100
Deutchman, D. E., 118, 122–23, 127, 134, 135
Development. See Human development
Developmental exchange among group members, 44–48, 98; and problem group members, 94–98; promoting, 46–48; sensitizing questions and, 65–66; writing themes and, 59–60
de Vries, B., 122, 123, 127, 135
Diaries, 108–10; as data in research, 123
Disability: adaptation to, 4, 16, 21
Divergent thinking: definition of, 81; in guided autobiography, 80–93; humor and, 81–82; metaphor and, 86–88; poetry and, 88–90
Divorce: adaptation to, 16; guided autobiography and, 3
Downie, N. M., 128, 135

Ebersole, P. P., 5, 135
Ego integrity: guided autobiography and, 5; reminiscence and, 14
Elbaz, R., 14, 135

Emotions: expression of, 27; in group process, 49–50; poetry and, 90; salient, 60–61. See also Humor; Tears
Empathy: guided autobiography and, 62–63
Erikson, E. H., 12, 135
Ethnicity: mental health and, 15–17
Ethnomethodology, 129
Exercise: therapeutic role of, 3
Existential enlightenment: as curative factor, 44–45
Expenses of guided autobiography groups, 42–43

Falk, J. M., 120, 126, 136
Family: contributions of guided autobiography to, 17–19; information about oneself from, 104–6; as theme of autobiographical writing, 69–70
Family legacy. See Legacy
Family reenactment: as curative factor, 44–45
Family tree, 105
Fisher, L. M., 118, 134
Food: breaks for, during group meetings, 43; memory and, 91
Fragrances: memory and, 91–92
Freedman, B., 127, 135
Frenkel, E., 127, 135
Freud, S., 123
Friendship: as outcome of guided autobiography, 2, 4, 54–55; therapeutic role of, 3; trust and, 45. See also Confidant
Fulfillment: guided autobiography and, 5; integration and, 6–10
Future orientation: guided autobiography and, 5, 7–9

Gardening: therapeutic role of, 3
Gaston, C., 124, 125, 135
Geering, B., 123, 134
Geiger, S. N., 130, 135
Gender. See Sex
Georgemiller, R., 5, 22, 135
Glaser, B., 5, 124, 135
Goals: as theme of autobiographical writing, 76–77
Goldwasser, A., 5, 135

Gordon, S. K., 5, 14, 134
Gould, R. L., 12, 135
Grandparenthood: storytelling and, 117–18
Greene, R. R., 5, 128, 135
Greenwald, A., 118, 122, 135
Grief, 48. See also Loss; Widowhood
Grotjahn, M. L., 44–45, 135
Group cohesion: creating, 30–35, 37; role of leader in, 27; sensitization and, 65–66; and size of group, 40
Group leader: co-leadership, 28–29; conquering group members' fear of writing, 82–84; coping with problem members, 94–98; creating the group, 30–35; ensuring institutional support, 100–102; goals for, 25–28; guidelines for, 23–44; promoting developmental exchange, 46–48; promoting group members' self-esteem, 11–12; role of, 17, 20–21; seat location of, 41–42; selection and training of, 29–30; self-disclosure by, 47–48; steps to being, 23–24; as timekeeper, 49
Group members: absenteeism of, 35, 39; cohesion among, 37; counterproductive, 94–98; creative expression in, 80–81; depression in, 98–100; dysfunctional, 34; goals for, 31–32; norms for, 35–36; problem, 94–98; recruiting, 33–35; screening of, 33–34; trust among, 45–48
Group process: counterproductive members and, 94–98; healing power of, 44–58; importance of, viii; mastering obstacles to, 93–102; outcomes of, in guided autobiography, 2; therapeutic factors in, 45; writing and, 57
Group rules, 35–36, 52–53
Guidance: as curative factor, 44–45
Guided autobiography: cognition and, 19; description of process of, 24–25; developmental exchange and, 44–48; goals of, x, 1; identity and, 10–14; isolation and, viii, 54–55; leading, 23–44; as a legacy, vii; meaning in life and, vii; next steps after, 103–13; older adults in, 3–4, 6; outcomes of, 1–22; overview of process of, 2–3; repressed memories and, 111–13; theoretical underpinnings of, 114–31;

Guided autobiography (*continued*)
therapeutic role of, vii, 3–4; two levels
of, 104–7
Guided autobiography group: cohesion
of, 37; cohort interaction in, 56; cost
of, 42–43; design of, 32–35; ensuring institutional support of, 100–102;
fostering participation in, 35–37;
goals for, 31–32; intergenerational
interaction in, 56–57; leading a, 23–
44; logistics of meetings of, 32, 37–
43; rules for, 35–36, 52–53; sharing
within, 45–46; size of, 36, 40, 93–
94; support given by, 18–19; types
of, 24–25
Guided autobiography process: anonymity and confidentiality in, 52–53;
creativity in, 80–93; humor in, 53–
54; sensitizing questions and, 63–66;
writing themes in, 59–63. *See also*
Group process; Meetings, group
Guided autobiography techniques: use of
food in, 91; use of metaphors in, 86–
88; use of music in, 90–91; use of poetry in, 88–90; use of puppets in, 92;
use of self-descriptive words in, 84–
85; use of sensual experiments in,
90–92
Guilt, 51–52

Hahn, M. E., 128, 135
Hall, G. S., 1, 123, 127, 135
Harkins, S. W., 5, 135
Hately, B. J., 5, 135
Hates: as theme of autobiographical
writing, 75–76
Havighurst, R. J., 5, 135
Health: as theme of autobiographical
writing, 72
Heart attack: use of guided autobiogra-
phy by victims of, 4
Hedlund, B., 5, 125–28, 130–31, 134
Hemingway, E., x
Heritage groups, 16–17
Hirn, K. F., 99, 134
History: use of autobiographical data in
writing, 120, 130–31; of autobiogra-
phy, 114–18
Hobbies: guided autobiography and
interest in, 4
Holt, R. R., 121, 135

Hope: as curative factor, 44–45
Hoppe, C., 9, 134
Hospice placement: guided autobiogra-
phy and, 4
Hostility: depression and, 100
Howard, R., 7
Hoyer, W. J., 116, 137
Hughes, J. A., 129, 133
Hughston, G., 5, 19, 135
Human development: ethnicity and,
16–17; guided autobiography and, 1,
4–22; subjectivity and, 122–23
Humanities: personal data and research
in, 130–31
Humor: creativity and, 80–81; in guided
autobiography process, 53–54

Iacocca, L., 116
Ideal self, 10–14
Identification: as curative factor, 44–45
Identity: construction of, 10–14; cul-
tural and ethnic, 15–17; developmen-
tal exchange and, 44–45; guided
autobiography and, ix, 84–85; self-
descriptive words and, 9–10, 84–86;
strengthening, through guided autobi-
ography, 9–17
Ingersoll, B., 2, 136
Insight: as curative factor, 44–45; guided
autobiography and, 62–63
Institutional staff. *See* Staff
Institutional support, 100–102
Integration, personal, 12–14; fulfillment
and, 6–10; guided autobiography
and, 5
Intellectual fitness: maintaining, vii
Intensive journal method, 109–10
Intergenerational interaction: benefits of,
56–57; guided autobiography and, 5
Isolation: guided autobiography and,
viii, 54–55

Journal writing, 108–10

Kahana, R. H., 134, 136
Kaminsky, M., 2, 21, 80–81, 136
Kastenbaum, R., 5, 14, 134
Kent, G., 122, 136
Kim, S. G., 130, 136

Klein, E. B., 127, 136
Knipscheer, C. P. M., 118, 136
Kohli, M., 120, 121, 128, 129, 133, 136

Leader. *See* Group leader
Learning: as curative factor, 44–45
Leary Interpersonal Checklist, 13–14
Leedy, J., 89, 136
Legacy: creating a, 110–11; family history as, 17–19; guided autobiography as, vii, 1; life themes and, 59, 63; publishing one's, 107; purpose of, 110; writing style for, 83–84
Lejeune, P., 115, 136
Levin, S., 134, 136
Levinson, D. J., 12, 127, 136
Levinson, M. H., 127, 136
Lewis, M. I., 2, 5, 128, 134, 136
Lieberman, M. A., 120, 125, 136
Life cycle. *See* Human development
Life-history method, 130
Life review: characteristics of, 118; consequences of, 4–22; definition of, 115; guided autobiography as, 1–2; techniques of, 2
Life satisfaction. *See* Self-esteem
Life themes: *See* Themes for autobiographical writing
Literary criticism: use of autobiographical data in, 120, 130–31
Loneliness. *See* Isolation
Loss: confidants and, 55; continuity and, 15–16; as theme of autobiographical writing, 74–75
Loves: as theme of autobiographical writing, 75–76
Lowenthal, M., 127, 136

MacLean, M. S., 128, 135
Maddi, S. R., 104, 136
Magee, J. J., 5, 19, 118, 136
Maloney, H. N., 5, 22, 135
Marxism: autobiographical data and research on, 129
Massarik, F., 5, 127, 134
McKee, B., 127, 136
McMahon, A. W., 98, 136
Meaning in life: continuity and, 14–15;

guided autobiography and, 5, 6; search for, 104–7; as theme of autobiographical writing, 76–77
Meetings, group: cost of, 42–43; format of, 39–40; logistics of, 37–43; seating arrangements for, 41; settings for, 41; times for and length of, 38
Members. *See* Group members
Memory: functioning of, 19; guided autobiography and, 1–2, 5, 111ʹ–13; poetry and, 90; senses and, 90–92; sensitization and, 64–65; writing and, 57
Mental ability: guided autobiography and, 5. *See also* Cognitive functioning
Mental health: cultural and ethnic identity and, 15–17. *See also* Adaptation
Merriam, S., 5, 19, 135
Metaphors: use of, in guided autobiography, 81, 86–88
Money: as theme of autobiographical writing, 71
Monopolizer, 95–97
Motivation: for autobiographical writing, 116, 119; effect of guided autobiography on, 19–20
Murray, H. A., 123, 127, 128, 136
Music: as theme of autobiographical writing, 77–78; therapeutic role of, 3; use of, in guided autobiography, 90–91
Myerhoff, B. G., 1, 5, 130, 136

Nehrke, M. F., 5, 14, 134
Nonparticipant, 97–98
Number Our Days (Myerhoff), 130
Nunnally, J. C., 122, 124, 137
Nursing: guided autobiography as tool in, 6
Nursing home: adaptation to, 3–4, 22; outcomes of guided autobiography in, 55; staff support in, 100–102

Occupation: correlation between, and autobiographical writing, 116, 119
"Oh" phenomenon, 51–52
Older adults: creativity in, 81–82; emotional frailty in, 27; group cohesion and, 37; group participation of, 35; guided autobiography outcomes for,

Older adults (*continued*)
3–10; interest of, in autobiography,
118–20; meeting times and, 38; reconciliation and, 5; roles for, 20–22;
social gains for, in guided autobiography, 54–57; thought processes of, 82
Olney, J., 115, 137
Oral history, 109, 117–18
Osterland, M., 129, 137
Outcomes of guided autobiography,
1–22
Overeating: depression and, 99
Overenrollment, 93–94

Personal data: accuracy of, 125–26;
analysis of, 125; current uses of,
126–31; methodological issues in use
of, 124–26; reliability of, 12, 122–
25; representativeness of, 121–22,
124–25; use of, in research, 120, 131
Personal growth: emotional support and,
50–51
Personality of autobiographers, 115–17
Photographs: use of, in guided autobiog-
raphy, 105–7
Planfulness, 19
Play: creativity and, 80–81
Poetry: use of, in guided autobiography,
81, 88–90, 108
Political science: use of autobiographical
data in, 120, 130
Power: as outcome of guided autobiog-
raphy, 4–5
Premo, T., 131, 134
Price, C., 17, 137
Progoff, I., 109–10, 137
Promotional materials, 30–31, 43
Psychology: behaviorism in, 120–23;
use of guided autobiographical data in,
120, 127, 128; guided autobiography
as tool in, 6
Publishing autobiographies, 107,
115–17
Puppets: use of, in guided autobiogra-
phy, 92
Purpose: guided autobiography and, 1;
self-esteem and, vii

Real self, 10–14
Recall: writing and, 57

Reconciliation: as outcome of guided
autobiography, 4–5, 22
Reedy, M. N., 13–14, 137
Relaxation: therapeutic role of, 3
Reminiscence: characteristics of, 118;
culture and, 117–18; definition of,
14, 115; guided autobiography and,
1–2; as play, 80–81; sensitization
and, 65; techniques, 2; writing
and, 57
Renaissance: autobiographical writing
during the, 115
Research: status of, in guided autobiog-
raphy, 114–31; uses of autobiographi-
cal data in, 120–31
Resolution: as outcome of guided auto-
biography, 4–5
Retirement: adaptation to, 16, 22;
guided autobiography and, ix, 3–4.
See also Transition
Rhudick, P. J., 98, 136
Riccio, A. C., 128, 137
Rich, S. L., 131, 137
Risks of guided autobiography, 98–100
Role change: adaptation to, through
guided autobiography, 20–22
Role clarity: guided autobiography
and, 5
Roos, J. P., 115, 120, 121, 129, 137
Rosenmayr, L., 129, 137
Rosenow, J., 129, 136
Runyan, W. M., 109, 124, 137
Ruth, J. E., 133, 137

Sarbin, T. R., 1, 137
Schafer, D. E., 5, 133
Schaie, K. W., 19, 138
Seating for guided autobiography
groups, 41–42
Self-actualization: emergence of, 11;
three versions of self and, 10–11
Self-awareness: guided autobiography
and, ix
Self-concept: creativity in, 84–85; metaphor and understanding, 86–88;
strengthening, through guided autobiography, 9–17
Self-descriptive words: creativity and,
84–85; identity and, 9–10, 84–86
Self-disclosure: guided autobiography
and, 5

Self-efficacy: three versions of self and, 10–11
Self-esteem: cultural and ethnic identity and, 15–17; guided autobiography and, 1, 5; humor and, 53–54; purpose fitness and, vii; and three versions of self, 10–11
Self-image, 10–14
Self-worth. See Self-esteem
Selling, B., 112, 137
Senior center administration: guided autobiography as tool in, 6
Senses: memory and, 90–92
Sensitization: group cohesion and, 65–66; memory and, 64–65; music and, 91; poems and, 89–90; reminiscence and, 65
Sensitizing questions: development of, 59; purpose of, 63–64; successful, 67–79; use of, in guided autobiography, 2–3, 63–66
Settings for guided autobiography, 32–33, 41
Sex: autobiographical writing and, 119–20
Sexual identity: as theme of autobiographical writing, 73–74
Shaffer, E. E., 125, 128, 137
Shute, G. E., 99, 137
Silverman, A., 2, 136
Size of group, 36, 40, 93–94
Sleep: depression and, 99
Slowing with age: creativity and, 82
Social acceptance: guided autobiography and, ix
Social-image self, 10–14
Social integration: guided autobiography and, 5
Social work: guided autobiography as tool in, 6
Sociology: use of autobiographical data in, 120, 128, 130
Speed of response: depression and, 99
Sperbeck, D. J., 137
Spiritual well-being: guided autobiography and, 5, 14–15
Staff: compliance of, with guided autobiography, 38; ensuring support of, 100–102; role of, in selecting group members, 33–34
Storytelling, 117–18
Stout, J. C., 131, 137

Strauss, A., 124, 135
Stress: as theme of autobiographical writing, 78–79
Substance abusers: use of guided autobiography by, 4
Suicidal thoughts: depression and, 100
Summers, H., 88–89, 137
Support, emotional, 48–49; guided autobiography and, 62–63; in guided autobiography groups, 36–37; personal growth and, 50–51

Tachibana, 92
Tears: depression and, 100; in group process, 49–50
Themes for autobiographical writing, 2–3; development of, 59; discussion of, in group, 39–40; emotional saliency and, 60–61; first, 61; importance of, 24, 59–63; order of, 59–60, 63; successful, 67–79
Therapy: guided autobiography and, vii, 3–4; referral to professional for, 35, 98–100
Thomae, H., 19, 123, 137
Thompson, P., 129, 137
Thurnher, M., 127, 136
Tolbert, E. L., 128, 137
Transcendence, 18–19
Transition: guided autobiography and, 3–4, 5; life themes in, 61–62
Trust: in group process, 44–58; tears and, 50
Tufte, V., 1, 5, 136
Tuvman, E., 128, 134
Tyler, L. E., 128, 137

Universality: as curative factor, 44–45

Vaillant, G., 54, 138
Videotaping guided autobiography, 84
Vocabulary: age and, 81–82

Wachter, P. E., 115, 120, 130, 131, 138
Weintraub, K. J., 138
Whitbourne, S. K., 116, 137
White, R. R., 127, 138

Widowhood: adaptation to, 16; guided autobiography and, ix, 3–4
Willis, S. L., 19, 138
Withdrawal: depression and, 100
Wolf, J., 129, 136
Work: as theme of autobiographical writing, 70–71
Wrightsman, L. S., 116, 118, 122, 138

Writing assignments, 25, 27, 39; fear of, 82–84; poetry as, 88–89; reading of, 38, 49; value of, 57. *See also* Themes for autobiographical writing

Yalom, I. D., 45, 138

James E. Birren, Ph.D., D.Sc., is director of the Borun Center for Gerontological Research at the Multicampus Division of Geriatric Medicine and Gerontology, and adjunct professor of medicine/gerontology, University of California, Los Angeles. Dr. Birren's career includes being founding executive director and dean of the Ethel Percy Andrus Gerontology Center at the University of Southern California and past president of the Gerontological Society of America, the Western Gerontological Society, and the Division on Adult Development and Aging of the American Psychological Association. Currently, he is a member of the World Health Organization's Expert Advisory Panel on Health of Elderly Persons. Dr. Birren has published extensively in the area of aging. He is series editor of the internationally renowned *Handbooks on Aging* and has over 250 publications in academic journals and books.

Donna E. Deutchman is assistant director of the Borun Center for Gerontological Research at the Multicampus Division of Geriatric Medicine and Gerontology, University of California, Los Angeles. Her recent publications include coeditorship of *The Concept and Measurement of Quality of Life in the Elderly* and a special issue of the journal, *Gerontology & Geriatrics Education,* entitled "The Feasibility of an Institute of Senior Scholars."

Designed by Ed King
Composed by G&S Typesetters, Inc.
in Galliard text and display.
Printed on 60-lb., Finch Opaque
and bound in ICG Arrestox
by BookCrafters.